Underground Health Reporter™

Little-Known Discoveries That Make a **Dramatic** Impact on Your Health

A Compilation of Health Reports from the pages of the Underground Health Reporter™ E-Newsletter

Think-Outside-the-Book Publishing LLC

Second Edition

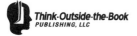

TABLE OF CONTENTS

Chapter 10   Healing: From Arthritis to Stroke

Chapter 11   The Healing Power of Your Mind

Chapter 12   Add Nourishment with Super Supplements

Chapter 13   Sexual Chemistry

INTRODUCTION

Practically every week, new health breakthroughs and alternative cures emerge that are proven to alleviate pain and suffering ... cure disease ... reverse aging ... and contribute to the health of mankind. But oftentimes, such breakthroughs and cures are systematically suppressed by the medical establishment and the pharmaceutical industry because they threaten the profits of those industries.

To this end, the *Underground Health Reporter*™ e-newsletter was conceived, and its maiden issue was broadcast on the Web on December 1, 2009. The e-newsletter was designed to be a weekly dose of little-known, cutting-edge—sometimes unconventional, and always startling—health information that can revolutionize your health or even save someone's life.

Since its first issue in 2009, the *Underground Health Reporter* e-newsletter has gained tremendous popularity as a leading health and wellness publication online, amassing hundreds of thousands of loyal readers and subscribers.

This book is a compilation of some of the most popular articles that have appeared in the e-newsletter issues, and it comes with a searchable index that enables you to easily find health topics that are of interest to you.

Part One consists of the "Did You Know ..." articles, which are the cornerstone of the e-newsletter's popularity. Part Two consists of noteworthy article contributions from *Underground Health Reporter's* partners.

After reading this book, should you wish to learn more health secrets and little-known health discoveries ... or subscribe to the Underground Health Reporter e-newsletter for free ... or participate in our health community where you can share ideas, opinions, personal experiences, and health resources relating to alternative health, we invite you to visit our portal website at www.UndergroundHealthReporter.com.

Wishing you the best of health,

Danica Collins

Editor, *Underground Health Reporter*™

PART ONE

Did You Know....?

Two Rejuvenating Herbs Used by the World's Longest-Living Man

Did You Know...

that the secret to his longevity was two revitalizing herbs, *ginseng* and *Fo-Ti*, which deliver the "elixir of youth" effect?

Li Ching-Yun, resident of the Kaihslen region in the province of Szechwan, was a Chinese herbalist, martial artist and former university professor who had the longest *recorded* lifespan in history. He lived to be 256 years old (1677-1933).

According to one account of Li's married life, when he was over 200, he had outlived 23 wives and was living with his twenty-fourth wife—a

woman of 60. A *New York Times* article published at the time of his death in 1933 reported, "Many who have seen him recently declared that his facial appearance is no different from that of a person two centuries his junior."[1]

According to the book, *Nature's Medicines*, "Li's longevity was due to his strictly vegetarian diet, his calm and serene attitude toward life and the fact that he used two powerful rejuvenating herbs prepared as teas."[1] One of the herbs was *ginseng*, and the other was *Fo-Ti*.

Ginseng is a sweet-smelling herb native to China, Russia, North Korea, Japan and parts of North America. Today, American ginseng is considered the most potent. Grown primarily in Wisconsin, American ginseng appears to offer the most powerful health benefits when compared with other varieties.

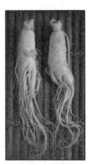

The herb is usually referred to as *panax ginseng* (panax is the Greek word for *panacea*, which means "all healing"). Ginseng roots are also called *Jin-chen*, which means "like a man" because they resemble the shape of the human body.

---

[1]Wilshire Book Company

Ginseng has been used as an all-around herbal remedy for more than 7,000 years, and it has been in widespread use since the eighteenth century. The herb's popularity has grown in recent years as scientific research studies showed ginseng's remarkable **health-enhancing and anti-aging abilities**.

Ginseng has been used successfully to treat a variety of medical conditions, including:

- *Memory Loss and Cognition Problems* — boosts brain function, especially in older adults
- *Diabetes* — contains active compounds that can help lower blood sugar naturally
- *Anxiety and Depression* — contains important *adaptogens*— natural substances that regulate the systems of the body—which help the body handle stress more effectively and alleviate anxiety and depression
- *Aging* — helps slow the signs of aging in most users
- *Dysfunctional Immune System* — helps boost the immune system and strengthen resistance to colds and flu, autoimmune diseases, etc.
- *Menopause* — helps relieve hot flashes and balance hormone levels, especially in perimenopausal and menopausal women
- *Chronic Infection* — strengthens the immune system so that the body is better able to fight infection
- *Chronic Fatigue Syndrome* — enhances the production of adenosine triphosphate (ATP) in the cells, thereby supplying the body with energy and relieving tiredness

Because of its wide variety of healing properties, such as natural blood thinners and immune system stimulants, ginseng is frequently used to fight cancer, diabetes and cardiac disease.

Fo-Ti, also called *he shou wu* or *ho-shou-wu*, is the dried tuberous root of the plant *Polygonum multiflorum*, an herbaceous climbing vine that is native to Japan. The plant is widely used as a folk remedy in China and other Asian countries. Fo-Ti should not be confused with the herbal mixture that is marketed as Fo-Ti-Tieng. Fo-Ti-Tieng is a registered trademark of a product that combines three herbs (*gotu kola* from India, meadowsweet from Europe, and kola nut, an African fruit, which is cultivated throughout the tropics).

Li Shizhen was one of the greatest physicians and pharmacologists in Chinese history. His major contribution to medicine is contained in his epic book, the ***Bencao Gangmu*** (*Compendium of Materia Medica* published in 1578). In that book, which was the result of 40 years of study, he described *ho-shou-wu* as follows:

> The root of the 50-year-old plant is called "mountain Slave": taken for a year, it will **preserve the black color of the hair.** The root [Fo-Ti] of the 100-year-old plant is called "mountain brother": taken for a year, it will bring a **glowing complexion** and a cheerful disposition. The root of the 150- year-old plant is called "mountain uncle": taken for a year, it will **rejuvenate the teeth**. The root of the 200-year-old plant is called "mountain father": taken for a year it will **banish old age** and give the power to run like a deer. The root of the 300-year-old plant is called "mountain spirit": taken for a year, one becomes an earthly immortal.

For over four centuries, the Chinese have regarded Fo-Ti as a reliable safeguard against old age. Fifty- to 300-year-old wild Fo-Ti plants are very rare these days; for the most part it is cultivated and collected after three to four years growth.

Perhaps Fo-Ti's greatest claim to fame is that it helps **maintain hair's original color**; that is, it *prevents premature graying and hair loss*. This is attributed, in part, to the herb's tonic effect on the kidneys and liver. According to traditional Chinese medicine theory, the condition of hair (on the head) is governed by the kidneys and nourished by the blood in the liver.

Age-Reversing Effects of Bee Pollen

Did You Know...

that many naturopathic doctors and health practitioners regard bee pollen as nature's "fountain of youth" because of its amazing age-reversing, disease-fighting, and health-boosting properties and super nutritional properties?

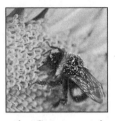

Bee pollen is a fine powdery substance collected by honeybees from the stamens of flowering plants, and stored in honeycomb hives. It is regarded by many as a *highly nutritious* and complete food—one which contains a rich supply of the B-complex vitamins and folic acid; vitamins A, C, and E; carotenoids; amino acids; some essential fatty acids; and a wide variety of minerals. Some nutritionists even insist that **a person can live on bee pollen alone**. This must be one of the reasons 10,000 tons of bee pollen are consumed every year by people all over the world.

Bee pollen's medicinal use dates back to the early Chinese and Egyptian societies where it was used for its **nearly miraculous ability to rejuvenate and heal**. Bee pollen was often entombed with Pharaohs, and the Romans and Greeks called bee pollen "the life-giving dust." Over 2,500 years ago Hippocrates,—the physician who is recognized as the father of modern-day medicine and one of the most eminent figures in the history of medicine,—favored bee pollen as a natural medicine useful in the battle against aging.

In 1975, Dr. Naum Petrovich, chief scientist at the Soviet Longevity Academy in Vladivostok, said, "Long lives are attained by bee-pollen users; it is one of the original treasure-houses of nutrition and medicine. Each grain contains every important substance that is necessary to life."

Bee pollen has been used to combat everything from cancer to weight management issues. Below is a partial list of its therapeutic benefits:

✓ Slows down and even **reverses the aging process**

✓ Super boosts the *immune system*

✓ Prevents and **inhibits the growth of mutated cells** that lead to diseases such as cancer

✓ Reduces *cholesterol, blood pressure*, and the *risk of heart disease* because it contains plant sterols and essentials fatty acids

✓ Relieves the symptoms of **Type 2 diabetes** by restoring mineral and energy deficiencies

✓ Fights bacterial infection the way antibiotics do

✓ Corrects and balances problems in the digestive tract and colon

✓ Supports weight management by **increasing the burn rate of fats and calories**

✓ Alleviates asthma and allergy symptoms by reducing histamines in the body

✓ **Eliminates cravings for alcohol and drugs** and removes toxins and contaminants from the body

✓ Relieves and rebuilds damaged, inflamed tissue (muscle and joint) through its extraordinary levels of antioxidants

✓ Combats fatigue, **depression**, and sleep disorders through its natural supply of "neuro-nutrients"

✓ Improves libido balance (over-undersexed) and enhances fertility

✓ Facilitates **cell generation and repair**, shortening the recovery time that result from exercise and injury

✓ **Enhances muscle mass and definition** because of its protein, iron, and vitamin content, which is higher than any other food and most commercially-developed muscle-building products,

Bee pollen reaches the mitochondrion level (where cell energy production and preservation occur), which gives it the ability to fight disease, heal the body, combat stress, reduce and reverse aging, and improve the skin's health and elasticity (less wrinkling and acne), to name a few of its effects.

Studies have confirmed bee pollen's life-prolonging, as well as its powerful antibiotic, antioxidant, and anti-inflammatory properties. When taken internally, it has been shown to immediately destroy dangerous bacteria that cause infection and disease, and **prevent the growth of cancer cells**.

Bee Pollen: A "Legal Sports Enhancer" Used by World-Class Athletes

Bee pollen has long been known to consistently produce more energy, vigor, and physical and athletic stamina in people who consume bee pollen as part of their daily diet. Athletes regard it as the *legal sports enhancer* because bee pollen contains as much as 40% protein, as well as all 22 amino acids. With almost twice the amount of protein as beef, twice as much iron as any other food, and substantial amounts of highly-absorbable vitamins and minerals, thousands of world-class athletes take bee pollen to give them a **competitive advantage**.

The British Sports Counsel saw a **40% to 50% increase in strength** of every athlete who took bee pollen regularly.

Most of our athletes take pollen food supplements. Our studies show that it significantly improves their performance. There have been no negative results since we have been supplying pollen to our athletes.

–Antti Lananki
Coach, Finnish track team that swept the 1972 Olympics

When most people start taking bee pollen, they immediately experience a significant increase in energy and a greater sense of well-being. Many have reported that over time, regular use helps alleviate various health disorders and retards the aging process.

The dosage recommended by many health practitioners for best results is between 500 to 1,000 milligrams a day. If you suffer from allergies, it is advisable to buy *local bee pollen* so that your body will build a defense to plants and allergens in your area.

Bee pollen can be taken in liquid form (extract or tea), capsule, chewable tablet, or as granules or powder that you mix into your food or drink. The taste is agreeable to most people—some say it's slightly sweet and has a nut-like flavor; others say it tastes like flour and honey mixed together. Granules are the most recommended form; many users start with one teaspoon a half hour before breakfast—with water, juice or milk—and gradually work up to two teaspoons a day. Children should begin by taking three granules and adding two granules per day to reach a maximum of one-half teaspoon daily.

Over 40 clinical trials show bee pollen to be a safe, powerful food supplement for people of all ages, including children, teens, and pregnant or nursing women.

WARNING: People who are allergic to bee stings are likely to be allergic to bee pollen. Before taking a full dose, try a tiny amount on your skin or the tip of your tongue to see if you experience any reaction. If all is well, happy buzzing!

Anti-Aging Benefits of *Goji* Berry

Did You Know...

that goji berries have been shown to promote longevity, reverse aging, inhibit cancer growth and provide a multitude of extraordinary healing benefits?

The ***goji berry***, or wolfberry, is a tangy/sweet, red-orange colored fruit that comes from an evergreen shrub found in temperate and subtropical regions of China, Mongolia and the Himalayas of Tibet. It is also known as *lycium barbarum, gou qi zi* or *fructus lycii*. It is considered by many to be the **world's most nutrient-dense food**—because it is rich in antioxidants, particularly ***carotenoids*** such as beta-carotene and zeaxanthin.

For over 6,000 years, goji berries have been used therapeutically and have been prescribed by herbalists in China, Tibet and India to:

- inhibit growth of cancer cells
- support normal liver and kidney function
- improve eyesight—protect against macular degeneration and cataracts
- restore libido and improve fertility
- strengthen leg muscles
- boost the immune system
- improve circulation
- promote longevity

In recent years, dried goji berries and goji juice have become widely popular—celebrities like Oprah Winfrey, Madonna, Victoria Beckham, Elizabeth Hurley and Mischa Barton, as well as many famous athletes and supermodels, are among their avid proponents.

Goji berries' popularity can perhaps be traced back to 2003 when Dr. Earl Mindell, R.Ph, Ph.D, MH, a leading nutritionist and bestselling author of *The Vitamin Bible* and dozens of other books, wrote a pamphlet in which he told the story of Li Ching-Yun, who lived to be 256 years old. Dr. Mindell attributed Li's longevity to goji berries, and called Li's story "a powerful testimony to [this] remarkable berry..."

In Asia, goji berries have been consumed for generations. They are considered the "longevity fruit," possibly because of their high antioxidant content. Foods high in antioxidants have been shown to **slow the aging process**. Antioxidants 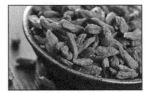 also eliminate the destructive power of free radicals, which helps to reduce the risk of many common, but serious, diseases, such as **diabetes**, high blood pressure, fever, and age-related eye problems.

One study, reported in the *Chinese Journal of Oncology* in 1994, found that 79 people with cancer responded better to treatment when goji was added to their regimen. Patients taking a cancer drug together with goji exhibited 250% higher recovery rate than patients taking the drug alone. The types of cancer that were shown to respond well to goji include malignant melanoma, renal cell carcinoma, colorectal carcinoma, lung cancer, nasopharyngeal carcinoma and malignant hydrothorax. Remission of cancers in patients treated with goji berries along with a cancer drug lasted significantly longer than those treated without goji.

Several other studies suggest that:

- Goji berry extracts may **prevent the growth of cancer cells**, reduce blood glucose and **lower cholesterol levels**.

- Goji berries have compounds rich in vitamin A that have anti-aging benefits. These special compounds help **boost immune function**, protect vision, and may help **prevent heart disease**.

- Goji berry extracts boost brain health and may protect against age related diseases such as Alzheimer's.

Goji can be an effective **aid to weight loss**. In a study in which obese patients were given goji juice twice a day, most patients lost a significant amount of weight. It appears that polysaccharides in goji reduce body weight by converting food into energy instead of fat.

Whole goji berries are sold at Chinese herbal shops. Most people consume the more readily available dried goji berries (shriveled berries that look like red raisins) and goji juice, which can be found in some health food stores (including Whole Foods) as well as online stores.

WARNING: There may be some drug interactions with goji berries. People who take anticoagulant drugs (also called "blood thinners"), such as warfarin (Coumadin®) may want to avoid goji berries. Goji berries may also interact with diabetes and blood pressure medications.

Maqui Berry:
A Modern Fountain of Youth

Did You Know...

that the Maqui berry *(pronounced mah' key)* may be a modern-day fountain of youth? This small purple berry, grown only in southern Chile, is considered one of the strongest antioxidants and is prized for its longevity-enhancing and anti-aging properties.

You may have heard about the benefits of drinking red wine in recent years. Now, consider this: Maqui berries give you up to **300% more anthocyanins** and nearly **150% more polyphenols** (the powerful anti-oxidants that give red wine its super immune-boosting power) than wine or any other fruit or vegetable known to man.

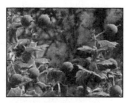

It's these high levels of anthocyanins and poly-phenols that give the berry its ultra-healing power. By providing the body with the antioxidants it needs, it frees the body of damaging free radicals that can actually cause premature aging and disease.

Since free radicals are the main culprit behind many chronic conditions and diseases—not to mention wrinkles and aging skin—it is no wonder that many people who take Maqui berry supplements are able to find quick relief from their aches and pains, enjoy vibrant health and look younger!

Some research has shown that taking Maqui berry decreases the recurrence of cancer in some patients. More studies are underway to discover exactly how effective Maqui berry is in treating and preventing cancer, but the initial findings offer a promising outlook for Maqui berry use in the treatment of cancer.

The polyphenols found in Maqui berries are known to protect plants from all kinds of infestations, and it is now believed that they are able to do virtually the same thing for humans. By protecting our bodies from the toxins and chemicals that bombard us on a daily basis—which may weaken both our skin cells and internal organs and systems—the Maqui berry can actually help to **rejuvenate cells, promote healthier aging** and even **ward off disease**.

What makes the Maqui berry so powerful? Many scientists believe it has something to do with the place where it grows. Found only in the Patagonia region of southern Chile and a small section of Argentina, the Maqui berry plant is subjected to a harsh environment and, as a result, must produce and store more phytochemicals to ensure its own survival. These higher nutrient levels are then passed onto the berries, and, when they are consumed by humans, they deliver this diverse array of health benefits.

Another important benefit of this super berry is its ability to control inflammation, which has led many arthritis patients to add it to their supplement regime, with wonderful results. Acting as nature's herbal COX-2 inhibitor, Maqui berries help to **reduce inflammatory responses**, which, in turn, helps to **decrease pain** and **increase flexibility and mobility**— even among people with severe arthritis and fibromyalgia.

Surprisingly, those who take Maqui berry regularly also tend to experience **considerable weight loss** as their bodies become healthier and able to dispose of toxins that may have been suppressing weight loss.

Maqui berry isn't just good for you; it tastes good, too. Unfortunately, it is virtually impossible to find fresh Maqui berries because they grow only in remote areas, which makes it difficult to harvest, store and ship to stores around the world, and the berries have a short harvest period (they are only available for picking once a year), which limits the supply.

Maqui berry supplements, however, seem to offer most of the benefits the fresh fruit does, which is good news for health consumers in need of a supplement that delivers these amazing benefits. Appearing on store shelves across America for the first time only about a year ago, it wasn't always easy to find Maqui berry supplements, but, today, most health food stores stock them all year round, as do many Internet retailers.

Cells Grow Younger
with Auxinon-rich Foods

Did You Know...

that certain foods actually make you younger?

In an article titled "Make Cells Grow Younger," Brown Landone, a twentieth century medical doctor who later became a leader of the New Thought Movement, reported on the nutritional effect of enzymes on rats:

Experiments were made on old decrepit rats. Their age corresponded to that of a man of ninety years. They were fed with 'immature food'—that is, food which had not finished growth, sprouting new stems, young leaves. The results were amazing. The old decrepit rats were transformed, and their bodies began to grow younger.

"At about the same time, other scientists discovered a root-auxin in plant roots. When they extracted this auxin from the tips of young growing roots, and pasted it on the edge of a leaf, roots grew even on the edge of a leaf. This is the **miracle of auxinon foods**—they induce growth after their own kind of activity. A root auxin will grow roots and a youth auxinon will grow youthful cells.

"Youth-growing substances from new growing sprouts will induce cells to grow younger. There is something in the chemical substance of a young growing auxinon which, when you eat it as food, **makes the cells of your body reproduce younger cells** instead of 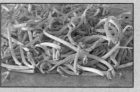 older cells... The best auxinon foods I know are produced in mung bean sprouts."

The No. 1 Longevity Food

Did You Know...

that the world's most incredibly sweet, decadent and satisfying food is actually good for you? Once considered the "bad guy" in the world of food, chocolate has turned into a national health-food phenomenon.

Chocolate comes from raw cacao seeds, the product of a fruit grown on the cacao tree (*theobroma cacao*). Cacao trees are exotic—growing naturally in the shade of tropical rainforests in South America and the West Indies. According to researchers, the raw cacao bean is one of nature's most fantastic super 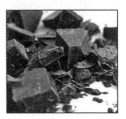 foods due to its mineral content and wide array of unique properties.

No wonder experts like nutritionist David Wolfe, author of *Naked Chocolate*, are extolling the benefits of the world's most popular comfort food. Its effects are far-reaching:

- Chocolate is good for *sufferers of asthma*, as it contains the anti-asthmatic compounds theobromine and theophilline.

- Cocoa, a component of chocolate, contains flavonels, antioxidants that increase blood flow to the brain.

- Cacao also contains high levels of sulfur and magnesium, which **increase focus and alertness**.

- Chocolate can actually **make you happier, longer** because cacao enhances the amount of time the happiness-inducing compound anandamide stays in your system.

- Chocolate **decreases anxiety and stress levels**. A clinical trial demonstrated that dark chocolate reduced the production of stress hormones in as little as two weeks!

- Chocolate is good for your teeth; the theobromine compound contained in chocolate **kills the bacteria that cause cavities**.

- Chocolate contains zinc, a key mineral that contributes to the health of your immune system, liver, pancreas and skin.

- Chocolate ensures your blood stays healthy, as it contains the key mineral, copper.

- Chocolate is considered by many nutritionists to be the **best food for your heart**. A study conducted by the German Institute of Human Nutrition found that chocolate consumption lowers the risk of cardiovascular disease, in part due to chocolate's ability to reduce blood pressure.

In addition, in a fifteen-year study involving men aged 65 and older, scientists studied the eating and exercise habits of 470 men—tracking their chocolate intake as well. Their results showed that, "The men in the group that *consumed the least* cocoa were twice as likely to die from a heart attack than those in the group that consumed the most cocoa." In addition, "Men in the study who *consumed the most* cocoa were less likely to die of any cause."

Just because chocolate is good for your health doesn't mean you should indulge in rich, high calorie, sugar-laden chocolates that are widely available. Many commercial chocolates contain ingredients such as refined sugar or unhealthy sweeteners, trans fatty acids and artificial flavors. The key to gaining the most benefit from the world's No. 1 longevity food is to choose chocolate that is:

✓ **organic**
✓ **dark** (not milk chocolate)
✓ **raw**
✓ stone-ground and/or **cold-processed**
✓ with a *minimum of additives*, which can negate the health benefits

Such chocolates are available at raw-food and natural-food stores, as well as online chocolate retailers like Sacred Chocolate.

The No. 1 Anti-Aging Food

Did You Know...

that chlorella is the world's greatest anti-aging food? It not only helps keep your skin youthful and wrinkle-free, but also helps you to live longer.

Chlorella is a single-celled, water-grown algae that contains more chlorophyll per gram than any other plant. It is extremely rich in vitamins, minerals, amino acids, essential fatty acids and many other nutrients that are beneficial to your health.

Chlorella also abounds in nucleic acids, which control cellular function and heredity. Two forms of nucleic acid are DNA (deoxyribonucleic acid) and RNA (ribonucleic acid). It is chlorella's **nucleic acid content** that gives it rejuvenating properties. Dr. 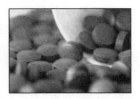 Benjamin S. Frank, author of *The No-Aging Diet and Nucleic Acid Therapy in Aging and Degenerative Disease*, found that nucleic acids promote the rejuvenation of the body's own DNA and RNA, enabling it to repair itself, utilize nutrients more efficiently, as well as remove toxins and produce more energy. Dr. Frank treated his patients with foods rich in nucleic acids, and reported that such a diet **made his patients look and feel six to twelve years younger than their chronological age**. They experienced a substantial fading of lines and wrinkles, and developed healthier, younger-looking skin after only two months of dietary nucleic acid supplementation (1 to 1.5 grams of nucleic acid per day) and a diet high in nucleic acids.

Of the nucleic acid-rich foods Dr. Frank recommended, *sardines* topped the list. He recommended consuming **one or two cans of sardines each day**, and claimed that his patients not only looked and felt more youthful as a result, but that they found it also alleviated health problems such as heart disease, emphysema, arthritis, memory loss, dimming vision and depression.

Sardines contain 1.5% nucleic acids, compared to red meat, which contains only 0.05%. According to the latest research by Dr. Minchinori in Japan **chlorella has seventeen times more RNA than canned sardines**. That's *exponentially more rejuvenating power* than Dr. Frank's sardine recommendation, which makes it the top anti-aging food.

Dr. Bernard Jensen, Ph.D., D.O. in *Chlorella, Jewel of the Far East*, reported that: Used regularly, chlorella would assist in the repair of damaged genetic material in human cells, protecting our health and **slowing down the aging process** ...When our RNA and DNA are in good repair and are able to function most efficiently, our bodies get rid of toxins and avoid disease. Cells are able to repair themselves and the energy level and vitality of the whole body is raised.

Chlorella is not just the top anti-aging food, it is a super food that has been used to treat some of the world's most devastating diseases including cancer, Alzheimer's disease and even AIDS. This all-natural healing food is believed to effectively reduce the symptoms of these and other chronic diseases:

- **Cancer**: Chlorella helps to accelerate the growth of immune cells and enables white blood cells to duplicate at a faster rate, which allows patients to better handle chemotherapy and radiation treatments. Chlorella has also been shown to have anti-tumor effects in some patients.

- **AIDS**: Because chlorella helps to activate T-cells and increase their reproduction levels, it has been successfully used to help thwart the onset of AIDS in some patients.

- **Alzheimer's/Parkinson's Disease**: Because it helps the body rebuild nerve tissue, chlorella has become an excellent treatment option for those suffering from degenerative brain and nerve disorders.

- **Viral Infections**: Chlorella helps give the body's white blood cells the superoxide they need to kill dangerous bacteria and viruses that make us sick.

- **Environmental Exposure to Chemicals and Poisons**: While not a disease per se, exposure to dangerous poisons and chemicals is fast becoming one of the major disease-causing factors. Chlorella appears to be a wonderful detoxifying agent that helps the liver clear out toxins and neutralize many poisons found in the body, including environmental poisons and toxic foods, thereby helping cells to rebuild themselves and repair damage that can cause illness and disease.

The phycocyanin found in chlorella also helps the body produce more stem cells, which is a great immune booster, and can actually be used to destroy bacteria and viruses within the body.

One of the stellar aspects of chlorella is its "growth factor," which allows it to **quadruple in size every twenty hours**—faster than any food crop on earth. This amazing ability is one reason chlorella works so fast at healing and repairing tissues and cells. Since it quickly multiplies the growth of good bacteria in the bowel, it is able to help the body eliminate dangerous free radicals more easily.

Most health practitioners recommend a starting dosage of three grams a day until the body gets accustomed to its powerful effects. Some people who use it therapeutically to treat more challenging ailments find that taking as much as seven grams a day helps them obtain the most benefit.

Turn Gray Hair
Back to Its Natural Color

Did You Know...

that regularly consuming fresh wheatgrass juice has been shown to turn gray hair to its natural color?

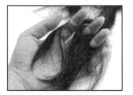

According to traditional Chinese medicine, hair pigmentation is influenced by the quality of a person's blood and the strength of their kidneys. Therefore, if your hair has gone gray, it indicates that your kidneys and blood need to be strengthened. Foods that accomplish this include wheatgrass and any food with high chlorophyll content.

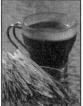

Wheatgrass is the young grass of the common wheat plant, *triticum aestivum*. Its leaves are juiced or dried into powder for human (or animal) consumption. It is often available in juice and smoothie bars, and is taken alone or mixed in fruit and/or vegetable drinks.

In *The Wheatgrass Book* by Ann Wigmore, she suggests that consuming wheatgrass juice acts as a beauty treatment that slows down the aging process because it cleanses the blood, helps rejuvenate aging cells and helps tighten loose and sagging skin.

The benefits of wheatgrass, however, go way beyond beautification and anti-aging. The high chlorophyll content of wheatgrass, as well as the amino acids, minerals, vitamins and enzymes it contains enable wheatgrass to provide a wide range of health benefits and curative benefits, such as the following:

- **Fights tumors:** Studies show that wheatgrass juice has a powerful ability to fight tumors without the toxicity that usually accompanies drugs.

- **Powerful detoxifier:** Wheatgrass protects the liver and the blood, and neutralizes toxic substances like cadmium, nicotine, strontium, mercury, and polyvinyl chloride

- **Protects the body against cancer cells:** Wheatgrass contains liquid oxygen, and cancer cells cannot exist in the presence of oxygen; and—is also vital to many other body processes.

- **Blood builder:** The chlorophyll in wheatgrass is remarkably similar to hemoglobin, the compound that carries oxygen in the blood. When the human body absorbs chlorophyll, it is transformed into blood, which transports nutrients to every cell of the body.

Note: Some health practitioners claim that you can double your red blood cell count just by soaking in chlorophyll. Renowned nutritionist Dr. Bernard Jensen found that wheatgrass and green juices are the most superior blood builders. In his book *Health Magic Through Chlorophyll from Living Plant Life*, he cites several cases where he was able to double the red blood cell count in a matter of days merely by having patients soak in a chlorophyll-water bath. Even more rapid blood building results occur when patients consume wheatgrass juice and other chlorophyll-rich juices regularly.

To learn more about this powerful superfood and seven other nutrient-dense superfoods that, when combined, create the 8-ingredient prescription for radically transformed health, go to: http://undergroundhealthreporter.com/the-8-ingredient-prescription-for-health/#axzz3FfIzt1TY

Chapter 2 - Cancer: Prevention, Treatment, and Natural Remedies

Simple Test Detects Cancer

Did You Know...

that there is a simple test that detects cancer anywhere in the body with a 95% accuracy?

Most people—and most doctors—have never heard about this test (called the Anti Malignan Antibody in Serum [AMAS] test). Many cancer screening procedures prescribed by conventional medicine are often harmful and invasive. Mammography, for instance, which is the most common procedure for detecting breast cancer, has even been shown to cause breast cancer. The National Cancer 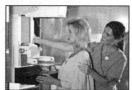 Institute (NCI) reported that, among women under 35, *mammography could cause 75 cases of breast cancer for every 15 it identifies!*

The AMAS test is one of the only known procedures for the early detection of cancer that is safe, non-invasive, and does not pose dangerous health risks.

> "Autopsy studies have shown that by age 50, almost half of all women have breast cancer, and 40% of men have prostate cancer." states Mike Anderson, filmmaker, medical researcher and the author of Healing Cancer from the Inside Out, and the film of the same name. Mike continues, "You can't prevent cancer. You're going to get cancer cells in your body. The average adult gets at least one cancer cell in their body every single day. And there's nothing you can do to prevent that from happening. The question is not whether you get cancer but whether your immune system is healthy enough to kill cancer cells and stop them from multiplying."

By the time you reach age 50, if you have, in fact, developed one cancer cell per day, you'd have 18,250 cancer cells in your body!

In 1974, Dr. Samuel Bogoch, a Harvard-trained neurochemist, discovered that as cancer cells collide with each other, their outer layer wears off, exposing the inner layer's "malignin" antigen. Clinical studies confirmed that the body perceives the malignin as foreign, and therefore launches a defense against the antigen with anti-malignin antibodies (AMAs).

Realizing that this discovery could provide a way to detect cancer in the body at the earliest stage, Dr. Bogoch devised a test (which later became known as the AMAS test) to measure the anti-malignin antibodies. Since malignin is related to most cancer cell types and locations, the test was *nearly foolproof* in detecting both common and uncommon cancers throughout the body including brain cancer, breast cancer, lung cancer, prostate cancer, kidney cancer, skin cancer, esophageal cancer, stomach cancer, anal cancer, thyroid cancer and 200 other types of cancer which affect millions of men, women and children.

Now, why would you want to undergo a test that could detect that you *might* have cancer? Clearly, it's because early detection affords you the lifesaving advantage of timely intervention and more treatment options.

The test kit is absolutely free from Oncolab, and it costs only $165 to have a world-class lab work through specific protocols to evaluate your blood sample for anti-malignin antibodies. The lab cost is covered by Medicare, and many health insurance companies will reimburse you for the cost. To find a lab, go to www.oncolabinc.com

Moringa: A SUPER FOOD that Prevents Cancer and Stops Tumor Growth

Did You Know...

that the super food known as moringa contains several thousand times more of the powerful *anti-aging nutrient* zeatin than any other known plant—and that it also has 2 compounds that prevent cancer and stop tumor growth?

The *moringa* is a genus of trees indigenous to southern India and northern Africa. It is a short, slender, deciduous tree that grows to about 30 feet tall. Once grown only in India, Africa and the Himalayas, it is now cultivated in Central and South America, Sri Lanka, Malaysia and the Philippines.

The leaves, flowers, bark, wood and roots of the moringa tree are used all over the world for a wide variety of pharmacological and nutritional purposes. But it is the leaves of the *moringa oleifera* species, in particular, that have recently become recognized as highly 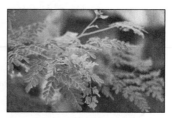 beneficial to human health. Compared with other green super foods like spirulina, wheatgrass and chlorella, *moringa oleifera* was relatively unknown until reports began appearing in mainstream scientific journals describing the medicinal and nutritional properties of these leaves.

Moringa, which is known as the "miracle tree" in many indigenous cultures, contains more than 90 essential nutrients. Practitioners of folk medicine as well as anecdotal reports suggest moringa's great value in reducing or retarding the growth of tumors. Studies show that two compounds present in moringa dramatically reduce the size of skin tumors and inhibit tumors in lab mice that have been bred to be susceptible to tumors. As a result, moringa has earned the reputation of being a **cancer preventative plant**.

Over the past 40 years, the World Health Organization (WHO) has been studying and using the moringa in third world countries where malnutrition and hunger are widespread because of its low cost and health-enhancing qualities. In India practitioners of natural Ayurvedic medicine use moringa leaves to prevent and treat over 300 diseases. **The leaves contain complete proteins, which is rare in the plant kingdom**, which is good news for vegetarians as well as for those who want to limit their meat and dairy consumption without compromising their protein intake.

A Bureau of Plant Industry report states that gram for gram, moringa leaves contain twice the protein content of eight ounces of milk (and four times the calcium); the Vitamin C equivalent of seven oranges; the potassium content of three bananas; three times the iron of spinach; and four times the Vitamin A of carrots.

Moringa leaves' rich combination of nutrients, amino acids, antioxidants, as well as anti-inflammatory and antibiotic properties could fill an entire book. But perhaps the most fascinating discovery about moringa leaves is that they are rich in zeatin, which is a member of the plant hormone family known as cytokinins, which induce cell division and growth, and delay cell aging. A study published in *Rejuvenation Research* shows the undeniable **youth-preserving effects** of zeatin on aging human skin, which explains why zeatin is becoming increasingly sought after. Zeatin defends cells against damage caused by free radicals, protects healthy cells from the effects of stress, helps the body replace dying cells more rapidly, and strengthens living cells thereby **slowing the aging process**.

No plant has a greater abundance of zeatin than the moringa plant. In fact, **moringa has several thousand times more zeatin than any other known plant**.

The human body contains approximately nineteen million skin cells at any given time. However, 30,000 to 40,000 skin cells die every minute. New skin cells make their way to the upper skin layers as the old skin cells flake off and die. The zeatin in moringa helps new skin cells grow at a faster rate than old skin cells die. This results in a **marked reduction in wrinkles** on the face and other parts of the body and a more youthful appearance.

Moringa dietary supplements are available as a leaf powder, leaf capsule and as a condensed powder tea.

According to Optima of Africa, Ltd., 25 grams of moringa leaf powder could provide the following astounding percentages of recommended daily allowances:

- Protein: 42%
- Calcium: 125%
- Magnesium: 61%
- Potassium: 41%
- Iron: 71%
- Vitamin A: 272%
- Vitamin C: 22%

For more information on how to incorporate moringa into your diet, go to: http://undergroundhealthreporter.com/moringa-health-benefits/

Cancerous Tumors Self-Destruct
with Brown Seaweed

Did You Know...

that an extract from brown seaweed has been shown to cause cancerous tumors to self-destruct, detoxify the body of chemical build-up and burn body fat?

The medicinal powers of seaweed have been known for centuries for their proven ability to *prolong life* and *enhance health and beauty*. Over the last decade, continuing worldwide research has shown brown seaweed to be the most beneficial of all seaweeds.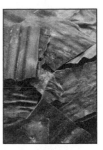

Brown seaweed (*Laminaria japonica*, or *kombu*) is rich in organic iodine, fucoidan, alginates, fucoxanthin, laminarin and other minerals. It also contains all of the 72 trace minerals, which people living in the Western hemisphere, particularly the United States often lack.

The following is a breakdown of brown seaweed's stellar health properties:

➢ **Fucoidan:** Approximately 4% of the total dry weight of brown seaweed consists of fucoidan, which is a sulfated polysaccharide, also referred to as an "evaporated oligomineral." It is the fucoidan content in brown seaweed that has been proven to cause certain types of rapidly growing cancer cells to self-destruct, according to the Biomedical Research Laboratories of Takara Shuzo and the Research Institute for Glycotechnology Advancement.

The phenomenon of **cancer cell "self-destruction"** is known as *apoptosis*, which is caused by a mechanism that is programmed into the nature of the cells themselves. When the apoptosis mechanism is triggered, the cell's DNA or genetic blueprint is rendered useless, and therefore destroyed. Apoptosis has been referred as the natural process through which living organisms expel harmful cells.

The health benefits of fucoidan have been documented in more than 600 scientific articles that can be found in The National Library of Medicine.[2]

---

[2]See http://www.ncbi.nlm.nih.gov/pubmed?term=fucoidan%20and%20cancer

The research shows that fucoidan's therapeutic properties include:

- immune system enhancement
- digestive/intestinal disorder relief
- allergy control
- liver functions improvement
- powerful anti-oxidant action
- cholesterol and blood pressure regulation
- blood sugar stabilization
- healthy skin and hair promotion

➤ **Fucoxanthin:** It is the fucoxanthin in brown seaweed that is credited with efficient fat-burning capabilities. However, fucoxanthin does not accomplish this by itself. Therefore, taking fucoxanthin supplements will not do the trick.

Fucoxanthin actually works in combination with the mineral iodine, which is also present in brown seaweed. When the thyroid is supplied with a sufficient amount of iodine, the endocrine system is rehabilitated and functions more efficiently, which—increases your body's metabolic speed, which allows your body to burn calories faster and prevent the accumulation of body fat.

➤ **Alginates:** Alginic acid, also called *algin* or *alginate*, is an anionic polysaccharide that is found in the cell walls of brown algae. The alginate content of brown seaweed detoxifies the body of strontium, uranium, mercury, lead, and hundreds of other toxic chemicals that we are exposed to in modern society. Such toxins, which become embedded in the heart, kidneys, liver, brain and other organs, are effectively eliminated from the body by sea vegetables, particularly brown seaweed.

Brown Seaweed Detoxifies Victims of Chernobyl

Perhaps the most convincing case study demonstrating the detoxifying ability of alginates in brown seaweed came in 1986 when the explosion of a nuclear power plant in Chernobyl, Ukraine enveloped the city and surrounding area in radioactive debris.

Modifilan, a super concentrated extract of brown seaweed, was rapidly deployed to people in all of the affected areas to help detoxify thousands of victims as well as more than 2,000 reserve-drafted men between the ages of 25 and 45, who were assigned the task of excavating Chernobyl and cleaning the sewage system. They were given about two tablespoons Modifilan daily for about two months under the supervision of doctors.

The results exceeded all expectations! In addition to Modifilan's ability to remove heavy metals from the body, those (particularly those over the age of 40) who had pre-existing health conditions experienced a wide array of health benefits. In addition, thyroid gland function was rehabilitated and the energy level of those who consumed the extract was increased.

> **Organic Iodine:** Most people think iodine is only important for thyroid function, but it actually benefits other organs as well as breast and prostate gland tissue. Many believe the rate of breast cancer in Japan is significantly lower than in the Western world is because the Japanese consume higher quantities of seaweed. A sufficient level of iodine keeps the thyroid functioning properly, and consequently regulates other glands and organs, including the pancreas, gall bladder, kidneys, adrenals, and even the liver.

> **Laminarin:** The laminarin content of brown seaweed is a great natural source of energy.

WARNING: Because of the publicity that brown seaweed has received in recent years, including a feature article in *Time Magazine*, it's not surprising that many people are heading to the nearest health food store and buying brown seaweed. However, there is a danger in simply buying brown seaweed in the form of kelp, or kombu or kombu powder as a dietary supplement.

Consuming large amounts of kombu can actually backfire because kombu consists of **indigestible cellulose or non-soluble fiber**. As little as a teaspoon of kombu powder, which appears finely ground, can feel like shrapnel to your colon because it is insoluble.

Diarrhea or constipation is likely to occur in those who start eating kombu in quantities larger than their bodies are accustomed to.

The extract of brown seaweed used in the aftermath of Chernobyl is manufactured by a company that hand-harvests the raw seaweed in the northwest Pacific, off the Kuril Islands, one of very few natural habitats in the world where wild brown seaweed grows to a size large enough to extract the viscous inner part of the leaves which contain the beneficial polysaccharides.

The outer part of the leaves is skinned off and put into a schnek feeder (similar to a meat grinder) and pressed through a tight mesh, thereby extracting a heavy gel and removing all heavy indigestible cellulose fibers. The batch of squeezed gel is then placed into a cold-temperature chamber dehumidifier, where it is quick-dried with cool air. As it dries, the gel hardens into a big rock-like chunk, which is broken into smaller chips, placed in a large grinder and turned into powder. This is Modifilan, which is basically the dried, concentrated juice of brown seaweed, which is fully digestible.

The company that manufactures *Modifilan* and *U-Fn*, the most bio-available fucoidan extract, does not sell directly to the public, but distributes its brown seaweed extract through a network of medical doctors, naturopathic doctors, dieticians, chiropractors, kinesiologists and other licensed medical professionals as well as online distributors.

Dissolve Cancer Tumors in Just 40 Seconds!

Did You Know...

that there is a hospital in China that routinely dissolves cancerous tumors using the 5,000-year-old healing practice called *Qigong*? In fact, a stunning videotape shows hospital practitioners dissolving an orange-sized tumor in 40 seconds!

The Huaxia Zhineng Qigong Center is the world's largest medicine-less hospital. Four Qigong masters from the hospital dissolved the tumor described above while two doctors monitored the procedure via real-time CT scan.[3] Since it opened in 1980, the Center has treated more than 135,000 patients with 180 different diseases—and has achieved an overall success rate of 95 percent!

---

[3]A videotape showing the cancer tumor dissolving in 40 seconds can be seen on YouTube at http://www.top10cancercures.com/registrationtop10.htm

Qigong (pronounced *chee gong* or *chee kung*) is a Chinese healing practice that employs movement, affirmations, breath work, visualizations and meditation to improve the flow of the vital energy or life force called *qi* (pronounced *chee*).

Qigong healing masters are able to heal a person simply by projecting qi on that patient—or that part of the body afflicted with the ailment or disease. In the early 1980s, Lu Yan Fang, Ph.D., a senior scientist at the National Electro Acoustics Laboratory in Beijing, China, discovered that the hands of Qigong masters emitted *high levels of low frequency acoustical waves*. Every human being generates such acoustical waves, but the signals generated by the Qigong masters are **100 times more powerful than those generated by the average individual**—and 1,000 times more powerful than those generated by the elderly or ill.

Qigong may seem unbelievable to Western doctors who are not trained in energy healing methodologies. However, Harvard physicians who have experienced Qigong healing admit they can feel electrical sensations in their bodies when a Qigong master projects his invisible healing energy onto them.

Dr. Hong Liu, a Qigong master now residing in California, and author of *Mastering Miracles*, has demonstrated the ability to project qi that is **lethal to cancer cells**. At Shanghai Red Cross Hospital, he emitted *qi* to kill cancer cells that were being cultured in a petri dish. The cancer cells in the dish died, while cancer cells in a control dish that received no *qi* continued to flourish.

Qigong has been shown to help heal not just cancer but also cases of HIV/AIDS, coronary heart disease, hypertension, digestive problems, asthma, arthritis, insomnia, pain, depression and anxiety.

Although the practice of Qigong takes years to master, there's a short-cut, "self-service" form of Qigong called Chi Lel, which is taught at the Huaxia Zhineng Qigong Center. It is a scientific and progressive self-healing system consisting of a set of simple exercises that dissolve blockages so that qi can flow throughout the body, bringing life to every cell.

One of these exercises is called *La Chi*. It is a simple and effective way to collect *qi* and use it to heal yourself or others. Many people who have come to the Center, and have been healed of cancer and other diseases, achieved those amazing results by using this *La Chi* technique. Here's how to do it:

1. Place your hands in front of you, away from your body, with the fingertips of both hands pointing at each other, almost touching.

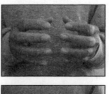

2. With your shoulders and hands relaxed, slowly move your hands outward until they are several inches apart. While doing this, imagine that your pain or sickness is leaving your body and disappearing into infinity.

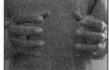

3. Move your hands back inward to the starting position until the fingertips almost touch. While doing this, imagine that you are directing qi or life energy to the part of the body where it is needed.

4. Repeat the outward and inward hand movements (Steps 2 and 3) for several minutes or more while affirming to yourself that all pain and sickness are gone, and that you're completely healed.

For more information, read *101 Miracles of Natural Healing* by Luke Chan, which explains the Chi Lel exercises more thoroughly and tells the stories of 101 individuals who miraculously recovered from cancer, diabetes, arthritis, paralysis, heart disease, severe depression, systemic lupus and many other chronic illnesses.

Fight Cancer Tumors with Olive Leaf Extract

Did You Know...

...that the phytochemical known as oleuropein found in olive leaf extract has been shown to eliminate cancer tumors in nine to twelve days?

It's no wonder that people who live in the area around the Mediterranean who consume twenty times more olive oil than Americans have half the incidences of cancer than people living in the United States. Both the olive leaf and olive fruit have active polyphenol properties, but in processing the fruit to make the oil, many are removed. Even so, olive oil contains enough polyphenols to deliver many healthful benefits.

Better than the oil is the **olive leaf**, which is prized for its antitumor, anti-microbial and anti-viral properties. The olive leaf comes from a small evergreen tree that is native to the Mediterranean region. Its medicinal use dates back 6,000 years. The olive leaf is even referred to in scripture as "the tree of life." Almost 2,500 years ago, Hippocrates— the acknowledged "father of medicine"—prescribed 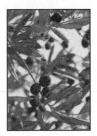 concentrated olive oil extracted from the olive leaf for numerous health conditions, such as muscle pain, ulcers and intestinal infections.

In our time, after four decades of research, scientists have identified *oleuropein*[4] as the substance in the olive leaf that accounts for its medicinal properties. Oleuropein is a phytochemical that contains one of the most powerful polyphenol antioxidants in existence, and has been shown to be a potent anti-cancer compound. Olive leaf extract contains twelve different antioxidants,—including hydroxytyrosol, which has an oxygen radical absorption capacity **ten times higher than green tea**, and tyrosol, which helps protect cells from injury caused by oxidation.

Olive Leaf Extract May Help Stop Cancer Dead in Its Tracks

Scientists initially believed that olive leaf extract had the ability to "cure" various diseases. But they later found that it actually does not cure disease directly—rather, it stuns or kills pathogens, which are disease-producing agents (such as a virus or bacteria). When the olive leaf extract interrupts pathogen activity, it essentially "unplugs" and "derails" disease in the making or inhibits the proliferation of disease in the body. Once pathogens are stopped dead in their tracks, the immune system can rebuild itself and "cure" disease at its root.

Some of the most amazing anti-tumor results were reported in *Biochemical and Biophysical Research Communications*. When oleuropein was administered orally to mice that had developed tumors, **the tumors regressed in nine to twelve days**.

The biochemists conducting the study reported that, "No viable cancer cells could be recovered from these tumors. These observations elevate oleuropein from a non-toxic antioxidant into a potent anti-tumor agent with direct effects against tumor cells."

---

[4]Oleuropein, a non-toxic olive iridoid, is an anti-tumor agent and cytoskeleton Disruptor. Hamdi K. Hamdi, Raquel Castellon at www.ScienceDirect.com

And it's not just cancer that olive leaf extract has been shown to treat successfully. Clinical tests conducted at the New York University School of Medicine showed that olive leaf extract was able to change the pathways of HIV-type infections as well, and may even reverse these conditions. In his book titled *Olive Leaf Extract*, Dr. Morton Walker recommends using olive leaf extract for its miraculous effects on more than 125 infectious and chronic diseases. Among its therapeutic uses are:

✓ Inactivation of bacterial, viral, and retroviral infections

✓ Prevention of dental and surgical infection

✓ Eradication of the HIV virus, as well as herpes and shingles

✓ Effective treatment for colds, flu and pneumonia

✓ Decrease in symptoms of Chronic Fatigue Syndrome

✓ Increased circulation, blood flow and reduced free radical damage (which helps combat heart disease, hypertension, and arthritis)

✓ Antifungal and antibacterial action on athlete's foot, mycotic nails

✓ Yeast infections

✓ Chlamydia

Studies show olive leaf extract is safe to take at therapeutic levels and has no side effects. It is widely available at health food stores in the form of capsules or tablets. The dosage will necessarily vary depending on the severity of the disease or health condition. As a rule, the higher the concentration of oleuropein in a particular product, the more effective it is thought to be. Dr. Walker recommends an olive leaf extract with an oleuropein concentration of at least 6%. Some brands have a concentration of 15% or higher. Consult with your naturopathic doctor to determine the dosage that is right for you. As a preventive measure, health professionals recommend one or two capsules equaling 250 to 500 milligrams.

WARNING: It is not advisable to use olive leaf extract in conjunction with antibiotics or other fungus or mold medicines.

A Mushroom that Cures Cancer and AIDS

Did You Know...

that the shiitake mushroom has been shown to be a powerful fighter of cancer and AIDS?

Over the past few centuries, the shiitake mushroom has been hailed as a botanical wonder with amazing medicinal properties. The countless benefits it provides have been supported by research and clinical trials conducted worldwide for many treatments involving cancer and the immune system.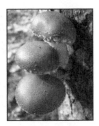

The shiitake mushroom grows on the wood of dead deciduous trees. Its medicinal use dates back to the Ming Dynasty (AD 1368-1644), where it was not only considered a delicacy, but it was also used as a remedy for upper respiratory diseases, poor blood circulation, liver trouble, exhaustion and weakness, and to boost energy. The flavorful mushroom was also believed to **prevent premature aging**.

Most of the formal studies of shiitake mushrooms have been conducted in Japan, where they have shown that an ingredient of shiitake, an activated *hexose containing compound* (also known as 1,3-beta glucan) has anti-cancer properties in humans as well as in animals.

Ever since the shiitake mushroom was shown to be a possible treatment for cancer and HIV infection, researchers in the U.S. and other countries have begun formal studies of the mushroom's medicinal properties. For example, the City of Hope National Medical Center is currently conducting clinical trials to determine if the shiitake mushroom can inhibit **lung cancer**.

In 1969, researchers at Tokyo's National Cancer Center Research Institute discovered a compound that they named *lentinan*. They found that mushrooms grown on logs have higher levels of lentinan than mushrooms grown on other types of organic material. Lentinan is a compound isolated from the shiitake mushroom, and is used as an **intravenous anti-cancer agent** in some countries.

Lentinan possesses **anti-tumor properties**, and human clinical studies have linked it with a higher survival rate, better quality of life, and lower cancer recurrence rate. Cancers that have responded well to lentinan include **colorectal cancer, pancreatic cancer, hepatocellular carcinoma, gastric cancer and cancers of the stomach**.

Shiitake mushrooms have also shown great promise in the fight against HIV. In some studies, the extract from shiitake mushrooms has proven to be **more effective in eradicating HIV** than azidothymidine (commonly known as AZT, the first antiviral treatment approved for use in the treatment of HIV). In a 1998 study done in San Francisco, it was found that patients with HIV infection who were given lentinan together with AZT maintained higher CD4 cell counts for longer periods of time than those who were given AZT alone.

Research has also demonstrated that the shiitake mushroom has the following therapeutic effects:

- Boosts the immune system
- Controls blood pressure
- Possesses anti-bacterial, anti-candida and anti-viral properties (including anti-HIV and Hepatitis B)
- Moderates blood sugar
- Enhances sexual potency
- Reduces stress

In addition, according to Japanese studies, shitake mushrooms contain a cholesterol-reducing amino acid known as *eritadenine*, which **lowers cholesterol levels by as much as 25% in one week**.

Once only a staple of Asian households, the exotic shiitake mushroom has found favor among the taste buds of Americans and others all over the world. They are now available throughout the year in many supermarkets across the United States. Shiitake mushrooms can be stir-fried or added to teas, soups or rice dishes.

For the best therapeutic results, many herbal medicine practitioners recommend taking extracts or concentrated forms of shiitake mushrooms at doses of one to three grams, two to three times daily. These products are available at health food stores and retailers of herbs and nutritional products. They can also be ordered by mail from online websites, including Amazon.com.

"Nutritional Chemotherapy"
for Curing Cancer

Did You Know...

that an extract of the turmeric root contains a phytochemical called curcumin, which has been shown to eliminate cancer cells?

Turmeric, the perennial herb which is prized in Ayurvedic medicine, is known to most of us as the gold colored Indian spice used in curry and mustard. Now, it is regarded by many medical practitioners as "nutritional chemotherapy." It is a low-cost, natural substance that countless people take every day to *prevent cancer*—and **at *chemotherapy* levels to treat cancer in early and advanced stages without side effects**.

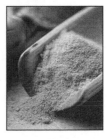

Curcumin is one of hundreds of constituents found in the root of the turmeric plant. People often use the words turmeric and curcumin interchangeably, but they are not the same thing. Turmeric is the whole food or whole herb; curcumin is an extracted component of turmeric—the one that has been singled out for its therapeutic properties.

Curcumin's medicinal use dates back 6,000 years to the ancient Egyptian pharaohs and Ayurvedic medical practitioners in India. Today, curcumin is used for its anti-inflammatory, antioxidant, anti-arthritic, anti-tumor and anti-amyloid (to combat neurodegenerative diseases) effects.

When curcumin's cancer-fighting properties were first "discovered" by Western medicine, an American pharmaceutical company tried to patent turmeric. Needless to say, health practitioners and suppliers from India were outraged since Indians have been using this herb for thousands of years to heal and treat major diseases.

Curcumin has broad anti-cancer effects during initiation, promotion, and progression of tumors. Several studies suggest that curcumin can cause cancer to regress ... has action against carcinogens ... substantially reduces the formation of mutagenic (cancer causing) chemicals ... and eliminates DNA damage to prevent the development of cancer."

–Karta Purkh Singh Khalsa (KP)

37

Yogaraj in Ayurveda, author of *Herbal Defenses*, and an expert on natural healing. Curcumin has been shown to be effective in both cancer prevention and treatment because it contains potent levels of:

> **Phytochemicals**: Non-nutritive plant chemicals that have protective or disease-preventing properties;

> **Polyphenols and chemo-preventives**: Compounds that actually block chemicals from getting inside cells and suppress tumor formation;

> **Antioxidatives and anti-carcinogenics**: Agents that act as free-radical scavengers, anti-mutagens, and bio-protectors that stop pre-cancerous and cancerous growth.

Curcumin is currently being targeted as a way to **reduce high breast cancer rates** because of its ability to slow and stop the division—and thus the spread—of cancerous cells. In a study on human breast cancer cells, **curcumin reversed growth by 98%**.

Another study demonstrated that using curcumin in mice successfully slowed the spread of cancer from the breast to the lungs, throat, and other areas.

Researchers at the University of Texas MD Anderson Cancer Center conducted a study that showed that when curcumin was added to cell cultures containing multiple myeloma (a type of cancer originating in bone marrow), it stopped the cancer cells from reproducing—and the remaining cells died.

Curcumin also obstructs cancerous cell growth by activating and protecting the release of human glutathione, which is a key antioxidant the body produces to maintain normal cellular activity and the only antioxidant that resides inside the cell. From this prime position, glutathione and curcumin inhibit cellular mutagens that would otherwise promote cancer.

Curcumin has also been shown to **reduce chemically-induced**—such as mouth and tongue cancer caused by smoking—**cancer by 90%**. Curcumin interferes with the process of the p450 enzyme in the liver that would otherwise convert environmental toxins into carcinogens, which mutate cells and promote cancerous growth.

Consuming fresh or dried turmeric root daily can help enhance your
overall health—but you would have to consume a staggering amount of
turmeric in order to experience curcumin's miraculous therapeutic and
health restoration benefits. Perhaps the biggest challenge in getting therapeutic levels of curcumin in the body is that curcumin is very poorly
absorbed by the body.

Studies have shown that the addition of the whole turmeric root full-
spectrum powder extract to curcumin with 95% curcuminoids, *significantly
increases the bioavailability of the active constituents* (i.e., the amount of
curcumin that is absorbed by the body).

When considering an over-the-counter curcumin supplement, it is
important to look for one that contains at least 700mg of curcumin extract
and whole turmeric root full-spectrum powder. Preferably, both curcumin
extract and turmeric powder in the supplement should be organic.

"Sunshine Vitamin" Could Eliminate
50% of All Cancer Deaths

Did You Know...

**that this nutrient could also prevent other diseases that claim nearly
one million lives every year?**

That nutrient is Vitamin D, the "sunshine vitamin," which is now
recognized by traditional and natural doctors alike as one of the most
powerful, inexpensive ways to prevent disease.

Vitamin D is found in small amounts in some foods, such as milk, eggs, fish, and fortified orange juice; however, the most important natural source of vitamin D comes from exposure to sunlight.

Vitamin D influences over 2,000 of the 30,000 genes in the body, which explains why it has been found to **inhibit the onset and spread of cancer**, heart disease, diabetes, multiple sclerosis, autism, rheumatoid arthritis, and osteoporosis, to name a few.

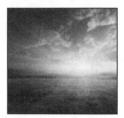

This common vitamin has the potential to help millions avoid some of the worst diseases on the planet, but people simply don't realize how critical vitamin D is to their body's normal cellular function. In the United States, Vitamin D deficiency is a public health crisis of epidemic proportion. Even those who are aware of the deficiency often do not fully understand the serious health implications that occur when the body's level of vitamin D drops.

After smoking, **not getting enough vitamin D is the No. 2 risk factor for cancer**! Every year, 50% of cancer sufferers worldwide—could be spared dying from cancer if they would just take the proper amount of vitamin D.

"Groundbreaking studies proved that **600,000 cases of cancer could be prevented every year just by increasing your levels of vitamin D**. And without question, the best way to obtain your vitamin D is by UVB sunlight falling on unexposed skin in doses that do not cause sunburn. Beyond cancer, increasing levels of vitamin D could prevent diseases that claim nearly 1 million lives throughout the world each year."

– Dr. Joseph Mercola, an osteopathic physician and
New York Times bestselling author of
The No-Grain Diet and The Great Bird Flu Hoax

When the body absorbs vitamin D, it converts it into a hormone called calcitriol, which the body uses to regulate cell growth and repair cellular damage, including malignant cancer cells.

Dr. Michael Holick, one of the world's most respected authorities on Vitamin D and author of *The UV Advantage* explains that "Vitamin D is made in the skin, gets into the bloodstream, and then goes into the liver and kidneys where it is activated into a hormone called 125-dihydroxy (calcitriol). It is this activated vitamin D that has biological, disease prevention effects, such as **preventing prostate cancer, breast cancer, ovarian cancer, and colon cancer**."

Thousands of dollars are often spent on health problems caused by a simple vitamin D deficiency. It can take months, sometimes years, of intense vitamin D treatment (i.e. 50,000+ IU's a day) to reverse the effects of disease.

The proper amount of vitamin D helps:

✓ Stop mutated cells from forming and spreading

✓ Cause diseased cells to commit "cell suicide"—make them literally self-destruct

✓ Cause cell differentiation (cancer cells are often undifferentiated, which causes them to reproduce faster than healthy cells)

✓ Reduce the probability that dormant tumors will regenerate into cancerous cells by inhibiting the growth of blood vessels in those areas

Absorption is the key. Dr. William Grant, Ph.D., Director of the Sunlight, Nutrition and Health Research Center, and an expert on the effects of the environment and diet on chronic disease, **recommends that adults get 2,000 to 4,000 IUs of vitamin D every day** from the sun or from vitamin D supplements to prevent cancerous or dysfunctional cellular activity. Most people get less than 300 IUs a day.

While it is possible with sufficient exposure to the sun to get 10,000+ IU's, there are several variables that inhibit the absorption of vitamin D, including:

- *Skin color* — darker skin needs 20-30 times more exposure than lighter skin to get the same amount of vitamin D
- *Sunscreen* — blocks the skin's ability to produce vitamin D by 95% (even when the sunscreen has a low SPF 8)
- *Weight* — overweight people absorb about half the vitamin D of normal-weight people
- *Clothing* — it is a myth that a little sun on the hands and face will provide enough vitamin D

- *Cloudiness* — cloud cover can filter ultraviolet B (UVB) rays, which are the type that converts into vitamin D (UVA are the rays that can cause cancer)
- *Location and time* — Seasons, geography (latitude) and time of day determine the amount of sun in any given place (for example, there is less sun in Alaska than Arizona, and less sun in winter than summer)
- *Fear* — that exposure to the sun will cause skin cancer

While it's true that *excessive* amounts of unprotected UVA rays can increase your risk of melanoma, a form of skin cancer, there is an overwhelming body of evidence that shows that *moderate* sun exposure combats cancer and other disease without risk.

It is virtually impossible to overdose on vitamin D. In fact, there's never been a reported case of vitamin D toxicity—so go outside and enjoy your daily dose of sunshine!

If you are unable to get sufficient sun exposure, taking a high-quality vitamin D supplement is recommended by many health practitioners. Natural vitamin D3 (cholecalciferol), or human vitamin D, is the type most often prescribed for therapeutic reasons because it is far superior to vitamin D2, which is synthetic.

Colloidal Silver: From Cancer Cells to Healthy Cells

Did You Know...

that colloidal silver has been shown to revert cancer cells to normal cells and kill harmful bacteria, viruses, yeast and molds in as little as four minutes?

Colloidal silver refers to microscopic particles of silver suspended in an aqueous solution, such as de-mineralized water. Technically, these particles remain suspended in the liquid for an indefinite period of time—without dissolving, or forming an ionic solution.

Low concentrations of colloidal silver (30 parts per million or less) are typically manufactured using an electrolytic process, whereas high concentrations (50 ppm or more) are usually either silver compounds or solutions that have been bound with a protein to disperse the particles.

The therapeutic use of colloidal silver goes back hundreds of years. It has long been taken internally to treat a wide variety of diseases. Before the advent of penicillin and the discovery of conventional antibiotics (methicillin, vancomycin, etc.), colloidal silver was one of the leading antimicrobial remedies. With the introduction of modern antibiotics in the 1940s, its use was discontinued.

A Suitable Alternative to Antibiotics

Antibiotics often cause symptoms to disappear, if only temporarily. On the other hand, antibiotics can leave a host of bacteria-resistant organisms, which may reappear at a later date and compromise the immune system.

A study conducted by Dr. Ron Leavitt of Brigham Young University (BYU) tested colloidal silver against antibiotics such as tetracyclines, fluorinated quinolones (Ofloxacin), the penicillins, the cephalosporins (Cefaperazone) and the macrolides (Erythromycin) on microbes such as streptococci, pneumonia, E. coli, salmonella, and shigella.

As reported in the *Deseret News* (May 16, 2000), Dr. Leavitt concluded that quality colloidal silver may serve as a suitable alternative to antibiotics. "The data suggests that with the low toxicity associated with colloidal silver, in general, and the broad spectrum of antimicrobial activity of this colloidal silver preparation, this preparation may be effectively used as an alternative to antibiotics."

In the 1990s, there was a resurgence of interest in colloidal silver as an alternative medicine. Since then, colloidal silver has been administered in different ways for specific purposes. It has been gargled, atomized or inhaled into the nose or lungs, dropped into eyes or ears, and used vaginally and anally. There is independent research on the use of colloidal silver in the treatment of cancer, hepatitis C, sinusitis, acne, yeast infections, flu, gangrene, colds, and other viral and bacterial infections.

Silver is a trace element that the body requires for good health. A deficiency of silver leads to a host of health problems. When silver levels are low or non-existent, for instance, cancer cells tend to proliferate. When a sufficient amount of silver is introduced, however, it safely and quickly kills the microbes inside the cancer cells, thereby **causing cancer cells to revert to normal cells**!

Colloidal silver also shows promise as a treatment for AIDS and herpes. In full-blown AIDS, the body's immune system is suppressed, making it susceptible to a wide variety of diseases. Colloidal silver offers a non-toxic supplement for 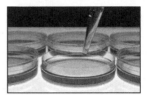 wide spectrum immune system support. Laboratory tests show that colloidal silver killed not only the Human Immunodeficiency Virus (HIV) in a test tube or petri dish, but it also **destroyed every virus, harmful bacteria, yeast and mold—in as little as four minutes**.

However, *in vitro* results (an artificial environment, outside the living organism) are not the same as *in vivo* results (in a living organism, such as the human body). The effect of colloidal silver diluted in a petri dish or test tube is significantly different from the same amount diluted in the five liters of blood—the amount contained in the human body.

It is important to note that colloidal silver only attacks harmful bacteria and pathogens, which are *anaerobic* in nature; it will not harm the "friendly" aerobic bacteria (such as lactobacillus and bifidobacteria), which the body needs. It does this by attacking the bacteria indirectly by disabling the enzyme that the anaerobic bacteria, viruses, yeast and molds require to survive, which *suffocates them*—without causing harm to human enzymes or the recipient's body chemistry. The result is the destruction of disease-causing organisms, including those that have become resistant to antibiotics. There is virtually no chance of bacteria developing resistance to colloidal silver.

Public concern about the use of colloidal silver erupted in December 2007 when a high-profile case of *argyria* became associated with the use of colloidal silver. Argyria is an extremely rare phenomenon that occurs when silver accumulates in the tissue under the skin, causing a blue or grayish tint—a cosmetic problem *not* a life-threatening one. What happened was that a Californian named Paul Karason consumed **gallons of colloidal silver** per week—for years. As a result his skin gradually turned blue. To put his case in perspective, the standard dosage is only one tablespoon per day—a far cry from gallons per week!

Argyria has only occurred in a handful of cases in the long history of colloidal silver usage. It is believed by many in the alternative health field that the hype surrounding argyria is nothing more than negative propaganda put out by "Big Pharma" to discourage the use of colloidal silver.

What do the pharmaceutical companies have against colloidal silver? We believe it is because colloidal silver is the only "natural" broad-spectrum germ-killer that can destroy virtually any known virus—including AIDS, H5N1 (Avian Influenza), SARS, Anthrax. If colloidal silver was widely used—not only could it potentially save millions of lives, it poses a threat to their earnings profits.

There are no known side effects from taking colloidal silver daily if you follow the manufacturer's suggested dosage or a physician's advice. Colloidal silver is sold as a dietary supplement in many health food stores and by online retailers. For those who want to make their own colloidal silver, generators and electrolysis equipment are available, which enable anyone to easily disperse silver wire into microscopic colloids of silver suspended in water.

Colloidal silver can be used topically or internally. For health maintenance and protection from colds, flu and other infectious diseases, a daily dose of one tablespoon is recommended. For existing infectious conditions, you might want to take one tablespoon three times a day; and as the condition improves, the dosage can be tapered down to two tablespoons a day, and, subsequently, to once a day.

For burns or sores, soak a cotton ball in colloidal silver and apply it on the wound using a bandage to keep it in place. This method has also been used to treat warts.

Many women suffering from vaginal yeast infection have received immediate results from a douche solution consisting of one tablespoon of colloidal silver mixed in with eight ounces of water.

Maitake: Case Studies Point to Amazing Cancer Cure

Did You Know...

that the maitake mushroom has been clinically shown to prevent and heal cancer, as well as decrease and even eliminate cancerous tumors?

Maitake (grifola frondosa) is a polypore mushroom that is native to Japan. It grows in clusters at the base of trees, particularly oaks, and has been prized for centuries for its medicinal properties. It is commonly known as hen of the 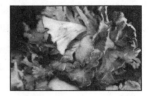 woods, ram's head and sheep's head; its Japanese name, maitake, literally means "dancing mushroom," a term derived from Japanese folk medicine.

Maitake is best known for its cancer-fighting properties. In 2009, a phase I/II human trial was conducted by Memorial Sloan-Kettering Cancer Center, which showed that maitake extract **stimulates the immune system of breast cancer patients**. The results of the study were published in the *Journal of Cancer Research and Clinical Oncology*.

Other laboratory studies involving Maitake D-Fraction (MDF), a standardized form of maitake mushroom containing *grifolan*—an important beta-glucan polysaccharide—show evidence of MDF's therapeutic value. It exhibits anti-cancer activity, has the ability to **block the growth of cancer tumors** and boost the immune function of mice with cancer.

The *Townsend Letter for Doctors and Patients*, Feb/Mar 1996 reported on a study involving 165 individuals with advanced cancer who used MDF in which this form of maitake was found **effective against leukemia as well as stomach and bone cancers**.

A Japanese clinical study investigated the effectiveness of administering a combination of MDF and whole maitake powder on 36 cancer patients ranging in age from 22 to 57 years old, who were in stages II to IV. **Cancer regression or significant symptom improvement** was observed in 11 of 16 breast cancer patients (68.8%); 7 of 12 liver cancer patients (58.3%); and 5 of 8 lung cancer patients (62.5%).

Here are just a few of the amazing case studies that show the immune potentiating effects of maitake in cancer patients.

> **Liver Tumor Disappears Completely:**

A 47-year-old female presented with Stage II hepatocellular carcinoma (cancer of the liver). In March 1994, she was treated with the drug cisplatin four times daily. In January 1995, she began taking maitake MDF and four grams of whole maitake tablets daily. The cisplatin treatment was discontinued. As of June 1997, the production of Interleukin-2 (IL-2) in her body multiplied by 2.2 times because of maitake administration. IL-2 is instrumental in the body's natural response to microbial infection. By July 1999, the tumor had completely disappeared.

> **Lung Tumor Vanishes and Doesn't Reappear:**

A 41-year-old female with Stage 3 intraductal carcinoma (**breast cancer**) had tumors that measured 2.4 cm and 0.7 cm in diameter. From September 1996, she underwent surgery to have the tumors removed, and then began taking ten mg of tamoxifen (TAM) and 100 mg 5-FU until December 1996. In June 1997, the cancer metastasized, and a 1.3 cm tumor was found in a lung.

She was then administered 125 mg MDF and four grams whole maitake tablets daily for twenty months. In March 1999, it was confirmed that **the lung tumor had disappeared**. While taking maitake, IL-2 production and CD4+ cells (a type of white blood cell that is important in fighting infections) increased by 1.5 and 1.3 times, respectively. As of early 2002, the tumor had not reappeared.

> **Stage III Cancer Turns to Stage I:**

A 45-year-old female with **Stage III liver cancer** had a serum bilirubin of 3.2 mg/dL, albumin of 2.1 mg/dL, and prothrombin activation of 43%. In May 1995, she began receiving transcatheter arterial embolization (TAE), 10 mL lipiodol (iodized poppy seed oil), 15 mg ADM, and 100mg cisplatin. This regimen was discontinued in January 1996 and was replaced by daily doses of 100 mg MDF and four grams maitake tablets daily, along with 100 mg of the chemotherapy drug 5-fluorouracil (5-FU). In February 1998 she began taking only maitake products and is now diagnosed as Stage I.[5]

---

[5]Noriko Kodama, PhD, Kiyoshi Komuta, MD, PhD, and Hiroaki Nanba, PhD., *Can Maitake, MD-Fraction Aid Cancer Patients?*

Case histories such as these illustrate the immune enhancing properties of MDF and whole powdered maitake. They also provide evidence that maitake has the potential to decrease the size of lung, breast and liver tumors.

Maitake is best known for its anti-tumor, cancer-fighting properties, but it has other disease-fighting properties, such as an:

> **Anti-Diabetic:** People with Type 2 Diabetes have been found to benefit from maitake mushrooms, which have the ability to lower blood sugar because they naturally contain an alpha glucosidase inhibitor. A specific, high-molecular polysaccharide called the Xfraction appears to be the active compound with anti-diabetic properties.

> **Anti-Hepatitic:** In clinical trials with 32 chronic hepatitis B patients, there was a 72% recovery rate in the group that was administered maitake, as compared to 57% in the control group.

> **Anti-Hyperlipid:** Many doctors in Japan use maitake mushrooms to 1) lower serum and liver lipids (such as cholesterol, triglycerides, and phospholipids) and 2) regulate blood pressure —two key risk factors in heart disease.

Maitake mushrooms are eaten raw or cooked. Many people consume maitake as a dietary supplement in the form of capsules and extracts called Maitake D-Fraction.

Warning: Canola Oil Linked to Lung Cancer

Did You Know...

that canola oil can be hazardous to your health and has been known to cause certain types of cancer?

The following excerpt is from *The One-Minute Cure: The Secret to Healing Virtually All Diseases* by Madison Cavanaugh, and is reprinted by permission:

> In 1986, canola oil was touted as a healthy oil because it is lower in saturated fat (6%) than any other oil. In contrast, peanut oil contains 18%, and palm oil, 79%.

Because canola oil also contains cholesterol-balancing monounsaturated fat comparable to olive oil, the Canola Council of Canada *attempted* to link many of the benefits of olive-oil-rich Mediterranean-type diets to diets high in canola oil—even if canola oil has never been used in Mediterranean cuisine.

The **propaganda** worked, and sales of canola oil have been on the upswing ever since.

However, not too many people know that frying with canola oil releases toxic, carcinogenic fumes. In recent epidemiological studies, it was shown that **high lung cancer rates** in Chinese women were linked to wok cooking with canola (also called rapeseed) oil. Consumption of canola oil has been shown to cause fibrotic lesions of the heart, CNS degenerative disorders, **prostate cancer**, anemia, lung cancer, constipation, irritation of the mucous membranes and many toxic effects, according to many nutritionists and biochemists.

A superior alternative to canola oil—and indeed the healthiest oil for cooking—is, and has always been, olive oil. Like canola oil, it's rich in monounsaturated fats, which help reduce "unhealthy" LDL cholesterol and boost "healthy" HDL cholesterol—without the toxic effects of canola. Olive oil also has a *high smoke point* (that is, the temperature at which a cooking fat or oil begins to degrade both the flavor and nutritional value of food), which makes it ideal for frying.

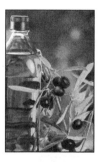

New research shows that virgin (and extra-virgin) olive oils—which refers to oils that are produced purely by mechanically pressing the oil from olives (i.e., no chemical processing)—are even more beneficial because they contain antioxidants called polyphenols. Polyphenols, which are found in olives, as well as red wine and green tea, mop up free radicals before they can oxidize LDL. Once LDL oxidizes, it becomes extremely damaging to arteries.

Chapter 3 - DNA: No Longer Destiny;
It *Can* Change

Change Your DNA Blueprint,
Create a Healthy Body

Did You Know...

that you can program your DNA to create a healthy body in as little as two minutes?

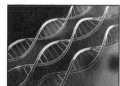

DNA is a nucleic acid that carries the genetic information in the cell. It is known as the "blueprint" of life because it governs the development and functions of humans and all living organisms.

It is a widely held belief that DNA, which is shaped like a double helix, has a *fixed* structure and cannot be changed,—but a recent study from the Institute of HeartMath has shed **startling** results that challenge what we *thought* we knew about DNA.

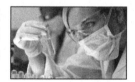

In the study, human DNA was placed in a sealed test tube. Test subjects trained to generate focused feelings of deep love were able to intentionally cause a change in the shape of the DNA.

Negative emotions, produced at will, caused the two strands that comprise human DNA to *wind more tightly*. Heart-centered feelings of love and appreciation generated by the research subjects caused the DNA strands to **unwind** and exhibit positive changes in **just two minutes**. When those feelings were absent, no changes in the DNA were observed.

This may be the first scientific evidence of the long-held theory that emotion greatly affects our health and quality of life, and is proof positive that we can communicate with our DNA through emotion—and thus, change the very blueprint of our health and our lives.

In her book *The Greatest Manifestation Principle in the World,* Carnelian Sage presents an **ingenious approach to producing deep feelings of love at will**:

Love is clearly something awesome embodying every person that is far greater than the genetic information stored in the DNA which resides in the nucleus of each human cell. Some refer to it as the vast intelligence that comprises our entire being, and some call it energy. Indeed, love is energy in its most fundamental sense—the raw material of all that is. **It's the most profoundly essential and transformative energy**, without which life itself would not be possible.

Indeed, if we can influence the behavior of DNA in a test tube, what untold health benefits might we experience by changing the DNA in our bodies through feelings of deep love? Perhaps that's what Carnelian Sage meant when she wrote, "Love and illness cannot coexist."

The Healing Power of a Single Musical Note

Did You Know...

...that simply listening to a single musical note that vibrates at 528 Hz has been shown to repair your DNA?

Western music is tuned to the Twelve-tone Equal Temperament Scale in which each note vibrates within certain limits. However, there is also an ancient six-tone scale of electro-magnetic frequencies called the original Solfeggio Scale. This scale, which was lost for centuries 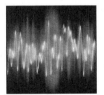 and was—by accident—just recently rediscovered by Dr. Joseph Puleo, is said to hold **unlimited potential for healing and personal transformation**.

One of the notes on the Solfeggio Scale, which vibrates at 528 Hz, has been **used by biochemists to repair human DNA**. The frequency of 528 Hz appears to influence the water molecules that surround the DNA helix, which, in turn, has a healing effect on DNA.

Perhaps the leading proponent of the miraculous healing power of the 528 Hz Solfeggio note is Dr. Leonard Horowitz, a Harvard graduate in public health and world famous author of fifteen books related to health science. According to Dr. Horowitz, **all healing is caused by sonic waves or vibrations**, specific frequencies of sound, resonating throughout the universe. He claims that human cells use DNA, like radios use antennae, to receive the note vibrations and attune the body's rhythm to that of the cosmos. He refers to the 528 Hz Solfeggio note as "the frequency of love" which, in addition to providing health benefits, opens the portals to *spiritual transformation.*

This view is echoed by Dr. Candice Pert, Ph.D., who states that energy and vibration go all the way to the molecular level each of which have 70 different receptors which begin to pulse in response to vibration and energy. This vibration, which happens at the cellular level, opens the chromosomes and exposes the DNA to the frequencies.

Experiments involving *in vitro* DNA exposed to recordings of different musical styles have been performed by Glen Rein of the Quantum Biology Research Lab in New York. Four styles of music, including Gregorian chants that use the Solfeggio scale, were converted to scalar audio waves and played via a CD player in a room with test tubes containing *in vitro* DNA. The effects of the music were determined by measuring the amount of UV light the DNA samples had absorbed after being exposed to the music for one hour. The absorption of UV light is regarded as significant because when the DNA helix unwinds, it allows such absorption.

The results of Glen Rein's experiments showed that the Gregorian chants caused a significant increase in the absorption of UV light whereas rock music had little or no effect. It was concluded that the audible sound waves of the Solfeggio scale can cause resonance in DNA and can, indeed, have profound healing effects.

To experience the effect of the 528 Hz note of the Solfeggio scale, just type "528 Hz" in YouTube.com and you'll find several videos that feature this healing frequency.

Spontaneous Remission: The Science of Thinking Your Way to Health

Did You Know...

that spontaneous remission from disease (including cancer) is now possible through the science of epigenetics?

A new field of science called epigenetics has changed the way we think about our genes. The prefix *"epi"* literally means *"above,"* as in *above the genes,* in the same way that epidermis means the layer above the skin.

Ever since Darwin published *On the Origin of Species* 150 years ago, science and medicine have been grounded in the belief that we are "programmed" by our DNA and that our genes cannot be changed. But new discoveries have revealed a *major flaw* in what was once dogma.

Dr. Bruce Lipton, a world-renowned leader in cellular biology and quantum physics research, proved that our **environment—not our DNA—shapes the development of our cells.** Dr. Lipton discovered that we have "epigenes" which attach to our cells and have control over the genes and DNA inside our cells. These epigenes change how our genes are expressed, which then changes our cells.

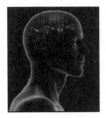 Dr. Lipton's experiments revealed that DNA responds to signals from outside the cells. Electromagnetic signals that are produced by our senses, thoughts, beliefs, and emotions as we experience the world send "messages" that reach the cells. As our minds constantly adjust to our environment, so do our cells.

These discoveries are being hailed worldwide as a major breakthrough that proves that **our bodies can be changed as we retrain our thoughts**. These findings fundamentally alter our understanding of life because if we can change our cells by changing our minds, we absolutely can change our biology ... and our lives.

Though our DNA is still considered the "blueprint" that we start with, epigenetics shows it can be altered throughout our lives. Think of your genes as the hardware and your epigenes as the software that tells the genes what to do.

Being able to change our genes offers a life-changing opportunity to the human race when it comes to the treatment of disease. No longer do we have to be a "victim" of inheriting or developing abnormal genes because we can now change them to eradicate disease and pass on normal genes to the next generation.

In one of Dr. Lipton's most important experiments, he took a "sick" cancer cell from a "sick" body, and transferred it to a healthy environment, and the cell recovered quickly and behaved normally. While working at Stanford University's School of Medicine between 1987 and 1992, Lipton found that changing the environment of cells made certain genes "turn on or off," which then altered the cell's composition, its health, and the traits

54

determined by that cell. These new constructions spread as the cell divided.

Based on his most recent work with cancer, Dr. Lipton has written that, "Genes are not controlling the life of your cells, **your mind is**. The mind and the beliefs that it holds—not defective genes—create a ripple effect that 'turns on or off' cancer cells."

Randy Jirtle, a geneticist in the Department of Radiation Oncology at Duke University, further explains that, "as our genes change, **cells can become abnormal, triggering diseases like cancer**. It's scary to think that a few changed genes can kill you. But it's also good news because we've traditionally viewed cancer as a disease solely stemming from broken genes. It's a lot harder to fix damaged genes than to rearrange your epigenetics."

Through epigenetics, **you can use your mind to "rewrite" your genetic expression**. You might, for instance, have mutated (diseased) genes, but you can rewrite their expression to normal. Disease treatment through epigenetics changes the structure of the cancer cell by rewriting the genes to act like normal human cells. In ongoing epigenetic trials, half the cancer patients are in complete remission.

Epigenetics works both ways: **your thoughts influence genetic expressions that can cure disease or cause disease**—depending on whether you have positive or negative thoughts, which are equally powerful. Therefore, you could have normal genes, and then through negative thinking express genes like cancer and other diseases. We see this in the "placebo effect." A patient suffering from a disease is given a sugar pill, but *believes* the "medicine" will be effective, and therefore, the person heals. Likewise, there is the "nocebo effect," which suggests that negative thoughts can not only make you sick, but can even kill you.

What's even more interesting, or disturbing, is that the thoughts and beliefs of other people, philosophies, cultures, and religions influence your perceptions, which then become part of your thoughts. Therefore, with whom and what you surround yourself can have a direct effect on your health!

Dr. Lipton says that, "you are innately able to heal yourself unless your perception says you can't. Since perception controls biology, whether you think you can or think you can't, you're right."

For more details on how to reprogram your DNA through Epigenetics visit: http://undergroundhealthreporter.com/reprogram-your-dna-and-cure-disease

Avocado: The World's Most Perfect Food

Did You Know...

that many nutritionists claim the avocado not only contains everything a person needs to survive—but it also has been found to contribute to the prevention and control of Alzheimer's Disease, cancer, heart disease, diabetes and other health conditions.

The avocado *(Persea gratissima or P. americana)* originated in Puebla, Mexico and its earliest use dates to 10,000 B.C. Since AD 900, the avocado tree has been cultivated and grown in Central and South America. In the nineteenth century, the avocado made its entry into California, and has since become a very successful commercial crop. Ninety-five percent of U.S. avocados are grown in Southern California.

The avocado, also called the alligator pear, is a high-fiber, sodium-and cholesterol-free food that provides twenty essential nutrients, including fiber, is rich in healthy monounsaturated and polyunsaturated fats (such as Omega-3 fatty acids), vitamins A, C, D, 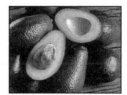 E, K and the B vitamins (thiamine, riboflavin, niacin, pantothenic acid, biotin, vitamin B-6, vitamin B-12 and folate)—as well as potassium.

Foods naturally rich in Omega-3 fatty acids, such as avocados, are widely acknowledged as the secret to a **healthy heart, a brilliant brain and eagle eyes**.

Dr. Daniel G. Amen, a clinical neuroscientist, psychiatrist, brain-imaging expert and author of the *New York Times* bestseller *Change Your Brain, Change Your Life* counts avocados as one of the top brain-healthy foods that can help prevent Alzheimer's Disease. That's not only because of the avocado's Omega-3 fatty acid content but also because it contains:

> ➢ **Vitamin E**: An international journal called *Alzheimer's Disease and Associated Disorders*, after years of clinical trials reported its findings that high doses of Vitamin E can neutralize free radicals and the buildup of proteins to reverse the memory loss in

Alzheimer's patients; reverse symptoms of Alzheimer's in the early stages and retard the progression of the disease.

> **Folate, also known as vitamin B9**: Helps prevent the formation of tangled nerve fibers associated with Alzheimer's. This water-soluble B vitamin also promotes healthy cell and tissue development. According to the National Institute of Health's Office of Dietary Supplements, "This is especially important during periods of rapid cell division and growth such as infancy and pregnancy. Folate is also essential for metabolism of homocysteine and helps maintain normal levels of this amino acid."

Below are just a few of the many more health benefits that the avocado's nutritional profile provides:

- *Monounsaturated Fats*: This type of fat helps control triglycerides in the bloodstream, lower blood cholesterol and control diabetes.

- *Lutein*: This is a carotenoid (a natural pigment) that protects the eyes against cataracts and reduces the risk of macular degeneration, the leading cause of blindness in adults 65 years of age and older. It also protects against certain types of cancer. Avocados contain three or more times as much lutein as found in other common vegetables and fruits.

- *Oleic Acid and Potassium*: Both of these nutrients help in lowering cholesterol and reducing the risk of high blood pressure.

You can add avocados to your diet in many ways:

1. The easiest way is to cut the avocado in half and sprinkle it with herbal seasoning or maple syrup.

2. Chop the avocado and add it to a salad, or use it as a topping or side garnish for soup.

3. Mash an avocado and spread it on bread or a bagel (in place of butter or cream cheese).

4. Cut an avocado in half and fill the hollow (left after you remove the pit) with your favorite healthy topping such as herbed rice or couscous.

5. Make an avocado dressing or the **crowd-pleasing guacamole** dip to add flavor to raw or steamed vegetables.

You can easily find many more avocado recipes online. Blended with fruit, avocados make a rich and delicious snack, side dish or dessert. They are also a highly nutritious baby food that delivers "good fat" for baby's brain and physical development.

Before you indulge in avocados to your heart's content, however, remember that because of their fat content they contain lots of calories.

According to WebMD, a medium-sized avocado contains 30 grams of fat, which is as much as a quarter-pound burger. That's why diet experts have long urged Americans to go easy on avocados in favor of less fatty fruits and vegetables. But now nutritionists are taking another look. They're finding that most of the fat in an avocado is *monounsaturated*—the "good" kind that actually lowers cholesterol levels. Thanks to this new understanding, the U.S. government recently revised its official nutrition guidelines to urge Americans to eat more avocados.

Coconuts: "All that Is Needed"

Did You Know...

that coconuts are one of earth's wonder foods? They can even save your life!

Few people (even fewer doctors) understand how important the coconut is to stabilizing blood sugar, lowering cholesterol, healing, hydration, and even **replacing blood plasma** in an emergency.

Referred to as *kalpa vriksha* (Sanskrit for "the tree that supplies all that is needed to live") in ancient India, and wherever they are grown, the coconut palm has been recognized as a top **immune booster**, *antifungal*, **antibiotic**, *antiviral* and **antibacterial** 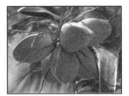 remedy for thousands of years. Yet, it has been only recently that modern researchers have begun to fully discover the *massive health benefits* this amazing fruit seed offers.

One example of coconuts' life-saving properties is their extensive use in the Pacific during World War II, when, because blood plasma supplies were scarce, it was very common for medics to siphon pure coconut water from young coconuts for use as emergency plasma transfusions for injured soldiers. Since coconut water is nearly identical to human blood, it was suitable for people of all blood types.

Because of its strong antioxidant properties, the coconut can be used to:

- Lower cholesterol
- Improve digestion
- Ward off wrinkles
- Stabilize glucose levels
- Fight off viruses
- Build cells
- Regulate hormones
- Increase thyroid production
- Lose weight
- Increase metabolism
- Fight infections
- Stave off memory loss
- Kill bacteria
- and more!

Because of its wide variety of uses, the coconut is one of the most treasured foods. Coconut products—including coconut flesh, coconut water, coconut oil, and coconut cream—deliver superb health benefits. Here are a few ways that you can use coconut products to stave off disease and to recapture the look and feeling of youth:

➤ **Coconut Oil**: Considered by many nutritionists as the best and safest oil to use for cooking, it is even superior to extra virgin olive oil when it comes to giving the body what it needs for optimum health. Unlike other fats and oils that we typically use for cooking and baking, coconut oil does not form polymerized oils or dangerous trans fatty acids, which can raise our cholesterol levels, clog our arteries and even make our skin sag and wrinkle. Plus, this ultra-safe oil provides important antioxidants that can help build stronger cells and improve your overall health and well-being.

In addition to being superior for cooking and baking, coconut oil makes a superb topical oil that can help to naturally rid the skin of dangerous toxins. It also gives the skin the perfect mix of hydration and antioxidants that it needs to stay healthy, smooth and younger-looking longer.

Another great benefit of coconut oil is in protecting your teeth from the bacteria that can cause cavities and disease. Simply rubbing a little fresh coconut oil on your gums and teeth can keep them stronger and healthier than virtually any other dental treatment.

Most people don't realize that coconut oil can actually help you lose weight! Yes, simply changing your cooking oil from any unsaturated fat to coconut oil can help you lose those extra pounds. That's because unsaturated fats found in canola, corn and other vegetable oils, as well as margarine suppress the metabolism, which makes it harder to lose weight —and easier to gain it. Over time, this metabolism suppression may result in 20 to 30 pounds of excess weight that your body cannot get rid of. Coconut oil, on the other hand, helps to increase thyroid function and boost your metabolism—essential to shedding unwanted pounds.

➢ **Coconut Water**: The coconut is a natural water filter. It takes almost nine months for a coconut to filter every quart of water stored within its shell. As a result coconut water is completely pure and sterile, which is one reason it can be used for blood transfusions.

Coconut water has the highest concentration of electrolytes of anything found in nature, which makes it an excellent source of hydration.

➢ **Coconut Cream**: The best skin treatment product you can use to achieve flawless skin may quite possibly be coconut cream. Unlike traditional skin creams which can actually introduce fats and oils to the skin that will break it down over time, making it look older, creams derived from the coconut can actually replenish the skin, giving it a more youthful look and healthy glow than most other skin care products on the market can.

When it comes to buying coconut products, coconuts are not all created equal. Wild coconuts are always best, but can be hard to obtain if you don't live in a tropical country. Whether you are using this wonder food to boost your immune system, increase your metabolism or fight wrinkles, using products made from young coconuts will help you reap the greatest benefit. Young coconuts contain the purer unsaturated fat than is found in the more mature varieties, and, therefore, offer greater rejuvenation properties.

You can tell how old a coconut is because young coconuts are usually green in color and oddly shaped. The brown hairy ones are mature coconuts, and while they offer a lot of health benefits, they aren't nearly as good for you as the younger ones.

Coconut-producing regions export coconuts all over the world so it's relatively easy to find coconuts at your local health food store, Asian grocers, and many supermarkets.

Hempseed: An Extraordinary Super Food

Did You Know...

that hempseed is one of the most nutritious food sources on earth?

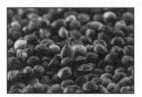

Without protein our bodies cannot repair cells, build new stronger cells, fight infection, build muscles, ligaments, and bone or even transmit messages from one part of the body to another. Most people, however, get their protein by consuming fatty meats and chemical-laden fish. Hemp, on the other hand, contains the highest amount of *edestin*, a plant protein that is constructed entirely of amino acids which can be used by the body to build important antibodies, enzymes, hormones, hemoglobin cells and blood-clotting agents.

Hemp also contains these vital nutrients:

➢ **Gamma Globulins**: These important antibodies are our first defense against infection and disease. Hemp is the world's best source of globulin-building materials.

➢ **Essential Fatty Acids (EFA)**: The human body cannot make these essential nutrients on its own; therefore, EFAs must be taken from the foods we eat. The challenge people face is that they aren't able to eat a sufficient amount of EFA-rich foods necessary to supply the body with the fatty acids it needs to function properly. Hemp is one of the few plants on earth that actually contains the ideal ratio of the essential fatty acids Omega-3 and Omega-6 (that is, a 3:1 to 4:1 ratio), which falls within the ratio recommended by the World Health Organization. EFAs are powerful antioxidants that protect our skin and cells from free radical damage, and they're also a great immune system booster.

➢ **Gamma-Linolenic Acid (GLA)**: GLA is an essential nutrient needed to fight inflammation and help balance hormones. GLA is difficult to obtain from other food sources.

> **Minerals**: The hemp plant possesses the ability to absorb a considerable amount of minerals from the soil. For this reason, it's an excellent source of major minerals and trace minerals, such as phosphorus, potassium, magnesium, sulfur, calcium, iron, manganese, zinc, sodium, silicon, copper, platinum, boron, nickel, germanium, tin, iodine, chromium, silver and lithium.

> **Amino Acids**: Hempseed contains eighteen different amino acids, including several detoxifying amino acids like cysteine and methionine, which helps the liver rid the body of potentially dangerous toxins.

With its wide array of important vitamins, minerals and enzymes, it's no wonder that hempseed is being touted as one of the best foods for both survival and sustenance.

Various hemp products are available via the Internet, but among them, hemp protein powder (which is also available in many health food stores) is perhaps the most important, especially for those who are protein deficient or who require high amounts of protein for body-building or other health pursuits.

Hempseed is also available in whole seed form, cold-pressed oil, hempseed butter, and a variety of products such as ice cream, chocolate bars, dressings, breads and even beer.

Oregano Oil: A Powerful Natural Antibiotic

Did You Know...

that oil of oregano's antibiotic properties have been favorably compared to streptomycin, penicillin and vancomycin?

Oil of oregano is pressed from the leaves of the oregano plant *origanum vulgare*, which should—not be confused with common oregano (*origanum majorana*) used as a culinary spice.

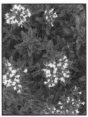

Although oil of oregano has long been prized for its *anti-microbial* and *anti-fungal* properties, and also as a remedy for stomach aches and coughs, recent studies have shown that its active ingredient, carvacrol, may be an effective treatment against bacterial infections that are resistant to antibiotics.

When used in low doses, oil of oregano has been favorably compared to streptomycin, penicillin and vancomycin when it comes to fighting Staphylococcus bacteria.

A study by Dr. Harry G. Preuss of Georgetown University, reported in *Science Daily*, confirmed that oil of oregano reduces infection "as effectively as traditional antibiotics."

The *Journal of Applied Microbiology* reported that among 52 plant oils tested, oregano was considered to have "pharmacologic" action against common bugs such as Candida albicans (yeast), E. coli, Salmonella enterica and Pseudomonas aeruginosa.

The issue of growing resistance to pharmaceutical antibiotics has been troubling to medical practitioners. Various germs have shown resistance to a number of antibiotics, including vancomycin, which is considered the most potent antibiotic. *Resistance does not appear to develop against a naturally-occurring antibiotic such as oil of oregano*. Pricewise, vancomycin costs approximately $16.00 per pill compared to approximately $1.00 for therapeutic strength oil of oregano.

Thymol, a chemical also found in oil of oregano, has been shown to be a powerful antifungal, antimicrobial, and antiviral agent. Many swear by oregano oil's ability to stop colds, sore throats and headaches dead in their tracks. Still others use the oil to get rid of nail fungi or athlete's foot. For best results, follow dosage directions on the package.

Oil of oregano is available in either capsule or liquid format at most health food and natural food stores as well as from online retailers.

The 60/40 Formula that Works Wonders

Did You Know...

green smoothies are a simple and healthy habit that is arguably the single most health-enhancing, weight reducing, healing, detoxifying and anti-aging habit you can adopt?

If you plan to make just one simple change in your life that can revolutionize your health, why not choose one that is among the best ways to **supercharge your body with energy** every day, cause you to **easily lose excess weight, detoxify your body,** slow down or even **halt your aging**

process, and **prevent and treat practically any disease**—all in one fell swoop? And it is easy to incorporate into your lifestyle and easy to stick to because it tastes so good?

The simple habit that can help you accomplish all this is *blending*—combining fruits and vegetables in a high-speed blender—and consuming the result in the form of a *smoothie* or *soup*. While this might not sound appetizing to those who are not fruit and vegetable lovers, the blends (also called "green smoothies") are actually quite delicious—even children like them.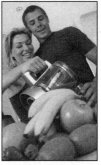

According to blending practitioners, the ideal fruit and vegetable blend contains 60% ripe organic fruit mixed with 40% organic green leafy vegetables. Some people add almond milk or soy milk to make the blend creamier. Green smoothies are often referred to as **the most nutritious meal on earth**.

Many advocates of blended food claim that when you include five fruits and three vegetables into your diet every day, it's almost impossible to develop a chronic disease. The human organism as a whole benefits significantly from the optimum nutrition provided by fruits and vegetables. Research shows that green smoothies can even **prevent and treat diseases such as cancer and heart disease**, and reduce one's risk of developing common health conditions ranging from age-related *cataracts* to *diabetes*.

The nutritional value of green smoothies has made them a trend that's gaining popularity not only among health-conscious individuals but among every day folk who seek to eat healthier, prevent or reverse disease, or fill in what's missing in their diets.

> Let your food be your medicine and
> your medicine be your food.
> – Hippocrates, the "Father of Medicine"

Blending "Green Smoothies" is Superior to Juicing

A juicer extracts the juice of fruits and vegetables, but discards the pulp into the waste chamber of the extractor. Even when one uses a masticating juicer that squeezes every drop of juice from the produce—leaving only dry pulp—that pulp, which is often discarded, contains one of the main

65

health benefits that comes from fruit and vegetable consumption—*fiber*. Blending **liquefies the whole fruit or vegetable**, thereby retaining the fiber in the drink instead of discarding it.

Many nutritionists believe that drinking juices extracted from vegetables with high sugar content (such as carrots) or from sweet fruits (such as dates, lychees and bananas) will spike the body's insulin levels, affect blood sugar levels and lead to an increased risk of developing diabetes and cardiovascular disease. That's not the case with blended fruits and vegetables, which retain the fiber, which slows down the release of natural sugars into the bloodstream.

High-powered blenders for green smoothies, like Blendtec and Vita-Mix, are able to break down the cell walls of the fruits and vegetables, thereby releasing all the nutrients which the body can readily absorb.

Another advantage of blending is that the green smoothies retain their freshness longer than juices. Although it's always best to consume smoothies as soon as they're blended, they can be refrigerated for up to a few days. Juices, however, begin oxidizing as soon as the juice has been prepared, and should, therefore, be consumed immediately. If they are not, the juice's nutritional content significantly deteriorates.

How Green Smoothies Can Help You Lose Unwanted Pounds

Glance at any list of the most common New Year's resolutions people make, and, invariably, you'll find that *shedding excess weight* tops the list. Diets can be difficult, but blending is easy, and it works.

One of the most riveting stories of weight loss I ever heard has to do with blending. A Costco employee named Clent Manich **dropped 240 pounds in one year** simply by consuming green smoothies daily. In the process, he was also able to beat Type II Diabetes and was completely off all of his medications and insulin within three weeks. His amazing story was chronicled in Victoria Boutenko's book, *Green Smoothie Revolution*.

Clent had made it a practice to start each day by making a gallon of blended fruits and vegetables so he could drink some of it every two to three hours. This helped **eliminate his food cravings** better than anything he had ever tried. Most other diets left him feeling hungry and weak. To get the exact recipe that helped Clent lose 226 pounds along with countless other smoothie recipies visit: http://simplegreensmoothiesolution.com

Here are just a couple of recipes Clent used to lose such a dramatic amount of weight:

> **Strawberry-Banana-Kale**:

    1 cup strawberries

    2 bananas

    1/2 bunch kale

    2 cups of pure or filtered water

> **Diabetic-Friendly Smoothie**:

    1 mango

    1 handful of blueberries

    1 bunch of dandelion greens

    1/4 teaspoon ground cinnamon (optional)

    2 cups of pure or filtered water

For additional green smoothie recipes and tips visit:
http://undergroundhealthreporter.com/green-smoothie-health-benefits

Recently, my friend Margo became an avid blending enthusiast after visiting her sister, Mallory, who saw that Margo was exhausted and clearly going through one of her bouts of depression. Mallory gave Margo a fruit and vegetable blend, and immediately after consuming it, Margo's energy level increased and her depression disappeared. That got her **hooked on blending**. From that day on, Margo made green smoothies every morning for herself and her kids. In a few weeks' time, without making any other changes in her diet, she had shed so much weight that she was able to *fit into her teenage daughter's jeans!* Margo, 49, and her two sisters (aged 53 and 55) had always struggled with the middle-age "bulge," but the green smoothies made their **excess weight melt away effortlessly**.

There are really no hard and fast rules for making a green smoothie, and you can vary the ingredients to make it taste the way you want it to—depending on what fruits are in season—while abiding by the guideline of using 60% organic fruits and 40% organic leafy greens.

The only appliance you need to blend efficiently is a high-powered, preferably commercial, blender for green smoothies. A regular blender doesn't have the power to liquefy or emulsify hard vegetables and fruits (such as carrots and apples).

Blendtec is considered by many green smoothie enthusiasts as the gold standard in quality blenders, and it's the one I prefer over Vita-Mix. Investing in a Blendtec or a Vita-Mix blender is well worth the investment for all the health benefits blending can give you and your family.

Parents use green smoothies to give their kids (as well as themselves) more vegetables and fruits in their diet that they normally wouldn't be able to consume in their regular meals.

Blended food tastes so good, both as a smoothie or a soup, adopting the practice may prove to be the easiest, healthiest and most pleasurable change you can make. And it is one that you can stick to. For dozens of additional green smoothie recipes visit: http://simplegreensmoothiesolution.com

Chapter 5 - Herbs: Add Spice to Your Life

Herbal Pain Killer: Better Than Tylenol?

Did You Know...

that there's an aromatic herb that relieves the pain of tension headaches just as quickly as aspirin and over-the-counter analgesics, such as acetaminophen (Tylenol)?

Tension headaches are the most common type of headache experienced by a vast cross-section of the population. Statistics show that 95% of women and 90% of men have at least one headache per year, and approximately one out of every six people in America experience the agony of chronic tension headaches.

As a result, most of us reach out for common over-the-counter headache medications, especially those containing acetaminophen, the most commonly used painkiller in the country today. On average, 7.3 billion adult Tylenol tablets are consumed annually.

But take heed: Each year, acetaminophen use causes **100,000 calls to poison control centers, 56,000 emergency room visits, 26,000 hospitalizations**, and more than 450 deaths from liver failure alone. Acetaminophen is a leading cause of acute liver failure, even at doses that are within the recommended range.

In May 2009, a U.S. Food and Drug Administration working group released a report urging stronger warnings and stricter dose limits for drugs that, like Tylenol, contain acetaminophen, and hence may pose an increased risk of liver injury if used improperly.

Given the risk, it is ironic that acetaminophen may not be the most effective way to stop headaches. That is because **headache pain does not originate from inside the brain**. The brain is incapable of feeling pain because it contains no sensory nerves. The pain actually comes from tension in the outer linings of the brain, the scalp and its blood vessels and muscles. Common tension headaches occur when the face, neck and scalp tighten up, and that tightening is often induced by stress.

Since headaches originate from the outer surface of the head, peppermint oil has been used to alleviate the pain. German researchers led by Dr. Hartmut Gobel conducted a randomized, placebo controlled, double-blind study that showed that **rubbing peppermint oil on one's forehead is just as effective in relieving headaches as taking a headache medication like Tylenol**.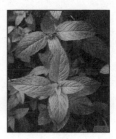

Confirming Gobel's results, in 1996, the leading headache researchers at the Neurological Clinic at Christian-Albrechts University in Kiel, Germany presented clinical proof that peppermint oil applied to the forehead indeed reduces headache pain just as effectively as the standard dose of 1,000 milligrams of acetaminophen (or two Tylenol tablets).

Researchers have long known that peppermint oil, whose main component is menthol, has an *analgesic and cooling effect when applied on the skin*. Menthol calms and soothes the excited nerve fibers in the painful region and can quickly make the pain subside.

Historians report that Gaius Plinius Secundus, better known as Pliny the Elder, a naval and army commander of the early Roman Empire, personal friend of the emperor Vespasian, and a writer and investigator into natural and geographic phenomena, recommended applying peppermint leaves to the forehead to treat headaches.

In addition to relieving headaches, peppermint oil has other therapeutic uses, including:

✓ Helping relieve gas, bloating, nausea, cramping and stomach upset

✓ Relieving muscle tension and pain by increasing the blood flow to the injured area, it aids in healing as well

✓ Alleviating stress

✓ Helping alleviate motion sickness

✓ Easing irritable bowel syndrome

Peppermint oil is available at Whole Foods and other health food stores.

The Power Herb that's Also
a Natural Aphrodisiac

Did You Know...

that the Peruvian herb, maca, is not only one of the best known natural aphrodisiacs, but is also highly beneficial to your health?

Maca (Lepidium meyenii), a hearty root vegetable belonging to the radish family, grows in the high Andean plateaus of Peru. It has gained the reputation of being a **super herb** in recent years, but it has actually been used for over 2,000 years to heal a variety of health conditions.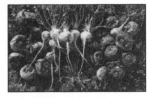

It is best known for its ability to enhance fertility and libido. Even before the Spanish conquistadors colonized the Inca Empire in the 16th century, the Incas had already been using maca for a multitude of health reasons.

In 1960, Gloria Chacon de Popovici, Ph.D., a Peruvian biologist, isolated the four alkaloids responsible for maca's reputed positive effect on hormonal issues such as **hot flashes**, fatigue, mood swings, memory loss—and even **male impotence**. Maca's reputation for restoring physical strength and libido has caused many a South American to nickname it "Spanish Viagra." (Note: Maca bears no resemblance to, nor does it have any association with, the trademarked drug after which it is nicknamed.)

Throughout its long history of therapeutic use, maca has been shown to:

✓ **Enhance libido and promote reproductive health**: The journal *Plant Science* reported that when maca was used in a reproductive health study, it **increased the sperm count in male test subjects in just two weeks!**

✓ **Alleviate the symptoms of menopause and PMS**: Indian women use it to treat menopausal symptoms, and Peruvian women have used it for years to encourage fertility and treat pre- and post-menstrual problems. Maca's calcium, silica and magnesium content helps prevent bone loss that may accompany menopause-induced osteoporosis.

✓ **Boost energy levels and aid in athletic performance**

✓ **Prevent certain forms of cancer**: Maca contains glucosinolate and fibers that help prevent prostate cancer and other types of cancer. In addition, its fatty acid content helps strengthen the body's immune system, thereby enabling to body to fight cancer.

✓ **Promote mental clarity**: Researchers have given maca to students before tests to improve their test scores.

✓ **Increase resistance to stress, trauma, anxiety and fatigue**: Maca is an adaptogen, a metabolic regulator that allows the body to avoid or heal damage caused by environmental factors.

✓ **Relieve pain and lower cholesterol levels**: Maca contains terpenoids and saponins which give it the ability to relieve pain, act as expectorant, sedative and analgesic—and even **lower cholesterol levels**.

Maca is rich in antioxidants, fatty acids, vitamins, minerals, amino acids and other nutrients that support optimum health. Because of its high iron content, it has been shown to be beneficial for those who suffer from anemia.

In Peru, maca is usually eaten like a potato, boiled and used in pudding, jams and drinks. Elsewhere, maca is more readily available at health food stores and from online retailers as a powder that can be conveniently added to food or drinks. Maca is also available in the form of capsules or liquid extract, both of which can be self-administered as dietary supplements.

To discover seven more of the world's most powerful superfoods visit http://undergroundhealthreporter.com/superfood

Cat's Claw: Miracle Herb from the Peruvian Rainforest

Did You Know...

that a tropical vine has been shown to be beneficial in the treatment of cancer, arthritis, AIDS, degenerative diseases—even premature aging?

Cat's claw, also known at *Uña de Gato*, is a tropical vine belonging to the coffee family that grows in the Amazon rainforest throughout Peru. The vine has curved, hook-like thorns that resemble the claws of a cat, thus the name.

Since the Inca civilization, South Americans have been using the powerful medicinal properties found inside the plant's bark to treat infections, arthritis, and gastrointestinal disorders.

Today, cat's claw is one of the best-selling herbs in the United States, for good reason. The inner bark of this "miracle herb" contains seven different alkaloids, concentrated tannins, and several phyto-chemicals that have been shown to be very effective in the treatment of disease as an: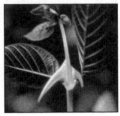

- ✓ **Anti-tumor agent**: Inhibits and combats the development of cancer;

- ✓ **Anti-inflammatory**: Reduces or inhibits inflammation that leads to arthritis and other degenerative diseases;

- ✓ **Anti-viral agent**: Treats viral infections such as HIV/AIDS

- ✓ **Antioxidant**: Terminates chain reactions that damage cells by removing free radical intermediates; inhibits other oxidation reactions that cause cancer, degenerative diseases, and premature aging;

- ✓ **Anti-microbial**: Inhibits the growth of microorganisms such as bacteria, fungi, or protozoans that strain the body's immune system;

- ✓ **Adaptogenic**: Rejuvenates and inhibits premature aging by building the body's resistance to stress, trauma, anxiety, and fatigue.

Many published studies by researchers in Austria, Spain, France, Japan, Germany, Peru, and the United States confirm the extraordinary medicinal uses of cat's claw.

For example, one of the seven alkaloids found in cat's claw, called Isopteropodin (Isomer A), contains a potent antioxidant that inhibits healthy cells from becoming cancerous. Procyanidolic oligomers—which are complexes of flavonoids/polyphenols that protect cells from destructive forces—have also been found in cat's claw. These inhibit the development and proliferation of tumors.

In addition, "five of the alkaloids have been clinically documented with anti-leukemic, anti-tumorous, and anti-cancerous properties. Italian researchers reported in a 2001 laboratory study that cat's claw directly inhibited the growth of a human breast cancer cell line by 90%." Separate studies found that cat's claw, "exerts a direct anti-proliferative activity specifically on the MCF7 breast cancer cell line," which reduces cancerous cell growth in that area.

Scientific reports dating as far back as the 1970s show that, "cancer patients taking cat's claw in conjunction with such traditional cancer therapies, as chemotherapy and radiation, had fewer side effects ... such as hair loss, weight loss, nausea, secondary infections, and skin problems."

Cat's claw is also considered to be a remarkably potent inhibitor of TNF (tumor necrosis factor). TNF is a cytokine (cell-signaling protein molecule) which causes cell death and tumorigenesis—a process by which normal cells are transformed into cancer cells.

Cat's claw was also discovered to be an anti-inflammatory in part because it reduces systemic inflammation through the suppression of TNF. It also contains quinovic acid glycosides, plant chemicals that have extremely powerful anti-inflammatory effects. Several studies indicated that, "cat's claw inhibits inflammation from 46% up to 89%. These results validate its long history of indigenous use for arthritis and rheumatism, as well as for other types of inflammatory stomach and bowel disorders."

In addition to benefits that it provides for the treatment of cancer and arthritis, cat's claw has been highly regarded as an immune system booster and as an anti-viral that has been used in the treatment of AIDS.

Many of these studies published from the late 1970s to the early 1990s confirmed that the immune-stimulating alkaloids in cat's claw increased immune function by up to 50%.

According to Michael Lam, MD, MPH, a specialist in nutritional and anti-aging medicine, "the alkaloids in cat's claw have a pronounced effect on the ability of white blood cells to engulf and digest harmful micro-organisms and foreign matter." Cat's claw increases the production of leukocytes and specifically T4 lymphocytes, which blocks the advance of many viral illnesses, such as AIDS. It also contains phagocytes which destroy viruses and other disease-causing organisms.

According to Dr. Satya Ambrose, N.D., cat's claw "enhances overall immunity while increasing stamina and energy in patients who suffer from physical and mental exhaustion due to an overactive or stressful lifestyle."

Cat's claw may be used as a preventative measure in people whose lifestyle is filled with constant stress and flight-or-fight responses that cause disease and premature aging.

Cat's claw can be taken as a capsule, tea, or tinctured extract. Dosages vary depending on desired effect. For example, the recommended dosage for osteoarthritis is 100 mg capsules per day and 250-350 mg capsules per day for immune support. Check with your doctor or naturopath for recommended doses in treating cancer, AIDS, and other health conditions.

Chapter 6 - Heal the Mind, Heal the Body

Deep Breathing: A Profound Healer

Did You Know...

that deep breathing is the single most powerful daily practice for advancing your health and well-being?

It might seem unusual, especially to people in America and the West, to regard the simple act of *breathing* as an activity that enhances health. That's because most of us think breathing is nothing more than an automatic, involuntary mechanism that we do to stay alive.

Special breathing techniques, such as those practiced in ancient cultures and certain Eastern disciplines (such as yoga), have remained largely a mystery to those of us in the West. What we often don't realize is that when we turn our 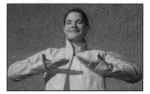 attention to our breathing—and increase the volume of air we inhale— beneficial physiological mechanisms are triggered that have a significant effect on health.

For example, when *volume, rate* and *attention* level are altered in the practice of breathing, **dramatic physiological, and even emotional**, changes can and do occur.

> The breath is a link to the most profound medicine that we carry within us. Within this nearly unconscious gesture, a breath, that we enact 1,261,440,000 (1 and 1/4 billion) times in our life span there is a **simple yet profound healing capability**.
>
> – Roger Jahnke, O.M.D., author of *The Healer Within*

Various advocates of breath work offer different breathing techniques and practices, such as full chest and abdominal breathing or alternate nostril breathing. The one I have been using since 1997 is one called Vital

Breathing. It involves inhaling, holding the breath, and exhaling in the following sequence:

- Inhale for one count

- Hold the breath for four counts

- Exhale for two counts

What's important is the **ratio** (1:4:2), not the actual number of counts that you inhale, hold your breath or exhale. For example: If you inhale for four seconds, then you would hold your breath for sixteen seconds and exhale for eight seconds.

If you repeat this breathing exercise ten times, three times a day (morning, evening and just before bedtime), for five to ten minutes a day, you will experience a noticeable shift in your energy level, your mental clarity and your body's ability to prevent and heal diseases.

One of the main reasons this breathing exercise delivers many health benefits is because the combined action of the lungs, diaphragm and thorax serves as a "pump" for the lymph fluid.

The lymphatic system is often referred to as the sewage system of the body. It cleans up the waste created by virtually all the other systems of the body. The human body has *twice as much lymph fluid as it has blood*. But unlike the circulatory system, which has the heart to keep the blood flowing, the lymphatic system does not have a "pump" to push the lymph fluids around the body. It relies on our **breathing** and **movement** in order to perform its function of surrounding every cell in the body; protecting each one by removing dead cells, blood proteins and any other toxins; and excreting them from the body. If the movement of the lymph were to stop entirely for 24 hours, you would die as a result of the trapped toxins and proteins surrounding your cells.

The practice of Vital Breathing creates the muscular movement required by the lymphatic system to circulate the lymph fluid efficiently. A lymphatic system that is functioning properly supports every other system in the body, including the immune, digestive, detoxification and nervous systems. A sluggish lymphatic system and stagnant lymph fluid, on the other hand, makes the body susceptible to infections, diseases and health conditions ranging from cancer, AIDS, tumor growth, cysts, impaired immune system—all the way down to cellulite.

> Improper breathing is a common cause of ill health. If I had to limit my advice on healthier living to just one tip, it would be simply to **learn how to breathe correctly**. There is no single more powerful —or simpler daily practice to further your health and well being than breathwork."
>
> – Andrew Weil, M.D.

The "Act of Kindness" Phenomenon

Did You Know...

that whether you are the giver, the receiver or the observer of an act of kindness—you reap tremendous benefits to your health?

This is a **phenomenon** that was discovered not too long ago. Numerous scientific studies have shown that kindness has a positive effect on the immune system and on the increased production of serotonin in the brain.

Serotonin is a *naturally occurring* neurochemical that has a calming, mood regulating, and anti-anxiety effect; it is regarded as a "feel good" substance because it serves as a pathway for pleasure in the brain. In fact, most anti-depressant drugs *chemically* stimulate the production of serotonin, which helps alleviate depression.

One of the most fascinating research findings to come out in recent years is that whenever a simple act of kindness is extended by one human being towards another, it results in a **significant improvement in the functioning of the immune system and increased production of serotonin** in both the recipient of the kindness as well as in the *person extending the kindness*.

What's even more amazing is that people observing the act of kindness experience a similar strengthening of their immune system and increased production of serotonin! Thus, kindness is a win-win-win scenario that produces beneficial effects in the giver, the recipient and the observer.

People naturally feel good when they give, help or serve others because they experience something called "helper's high," which Allan Luks and Peggy Payne, authors of *The Healing Power of Doing Good*, describe as a

feeling of exhilaration and burst of energy similar to the endorphin-based **euphoria** experienced after intense exercise followed by a period of calmness and serenity.

The benefits of kindness are not limited to immune system strengthening and serotonin production. Research has shown that those who routinely engage in acts of kindness, such as volunteers, experience alleviation of stress, chronic pain, and even insomnia.

In an article in *Psychology Today* (2/18/10) titled "What We Get When We Give" by Christine Carter, PhD states: People who volunteer tend to experience fewer aches and pains. Giving help to others protects overall health **twice as much as aspirin protects against heart disease**. People 55 and older who volunteer for two or more organizations have an impressive **44% lower likelihood of dying**—and that's after sifting out every other contributing factor, including physical health, exercise, gender, habits like smoking, marital status, and many more. This is a stronger effect than exercising four times a week or going to church.

A study conducted at Harvard University, called this phenomenon the "Mother Teresa Effect." Researchers showed a film about Mother Teresa's work among the poor people of Calcutta to 132 Harvard students. They 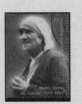 then measured the level of Immunoglobin A present in their saliva. Immunoglobin A is an antibody that plays a critical role in immunity.

The test revealed markedly increased levels of *Immunoglobin A* in all the test subjects—this, after simply witnessing a film of someone involved in charity work.

Considering the abundance of proof that acts of kindness increase one's sense of self-worth; enhance feelings of joyfulness; boost one's sense of physical and emotional well-being; increase one's sense of happiness, optimism and self-worth; decrease feelings of depression; and diminish the effect of diseases and disorders, it is clear that one of the best things we can do is find opportunities to extend kindness, and teach children to do the same.

Here are a few suggestions:

- Smile at strangers—especially those who are having a bad day
- Volunteer your time to do charity work or help wherever there is need
- Watch movies that display kindness
- Write a note to let someone know they are loved
- Pay compliments often
- Give up your place in line to another person
- Donate blood
- Write a thank-you note, especially to someone who's not expecting thanks

In their book, Luks and Payne state that volunteering, entertaining, regular club attendance, or faith group attendance is "the equivalent of *getting a college degree or more than doubling your income.*"

Six-Minute Antidote for Stress

Did You Know...

that there's an instant antidote to stress that you can do in six minutes?

If you turn on the TV, radio or the Internet these days, you're hit with **depressing** news about the economy, double-digit unemployment, the alarming numbers of foreclosures and bank failures.

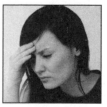

On top of that, you may also be overwhelmed by stress caused by your personal circumstances—a job you hate (or a job you're in danger of losing soon), a **demanding** boss, **messy** relationships, stacks of **unpaid bills**, tight **deadlines**, **plummeting** income and rising expenses.

WARNING: Don't ignore the stress that is present in your everyday life. Scientists have discovered that *everyday stress* is a factor for the **growth of cancerous tumors**, is a major **cause of heart disease**, and causes **your immune system to shut down**—making you susceptible to becoming a victim of any and all diseases. However you look at it, **stress kills!**

Dr. Alex Loyd has designed a revolutionary—and **free**—healing technique called *The 6-Minute Antidote to Stress* which **gets rid of the real cause of stress**. This simple technique, which you can do anytime—at home, at work or anywhere—neutralizes everyday stress, and instantly **rejuvenates** and **revitalizes** you in six minutes so you can:

- Function more effectively throughout the day

- Improve your outlook on life

- Sleep more restfully at night

- Enjoy better health—and *free* yourself from stress-induced diseases **no matter what your personal circumstances are**!

Boost Your IQ in Just Ten Minutes

Did You Know...

that you can become more intelligent just by listening to the "right" music?

A study was conducted by psychologists at the University of California at Irvine to determine the effect of specific kinds of music. The psychologists observed that participants who listened to ten minutes of Mozart's Sonata for Two Pianos (K. 488) achieved significantly higher scores on a test of abstract and spatial intelligence than participants who took the test without having listened to the music. They also found that when the participants listened to other types of music—a highly rhythmic dance piece or a hypnotic piece—there was no noticeable improvement in mental skills.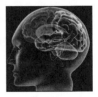

The UC Irvine experimenters also determined that people who listened to ten minutes to the Mozart piece before taking the test also did significantly better than those who listened to ten minutes of relaxation instruction or who sat in silence for ten minutes.

This phenomenon suggests that the complex musical composition typical of Mozart's sonatas **stimulate neural pathways** that are directly connected to mental skills. There is a growing body of science that asserts that music has a direct effect on human intelligence. For example, in an issue of Neurological Research, Rauscher and Shaw reported that pre-schoolers who studied piano **performed 34% better in tests of spatial and temporal reasoning ability** than preschoolers who spent the same amount of time learning to use computers.

Compilations of pieces by Mozart have been recorded on compact discs available to the public for the precise purpose of increasing IQ and achieving the kind of measurable IQ boost documented in this famous University of California at Irvine study.

Alzheimer's Disease:
Risk Factors & Prevention

Did You Know...

that *abstaining from alcohol* may actually increase your likelihood of Alzheimer's Disease?

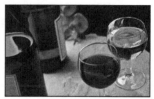

According to a seventeen-year study headed by Dr. Severine Sabia, and published in the *American Journal of Epidemiology*, drinking in moderation may help prevent Alzheimer's Disease.

Have you ever walked into a room and not remembered why you went into it? Losing your memory is a terrifying thing. Even if we joke about it and call our forgetfulness "a senior moment," memory loss, dementia and Alzheimer's Disease are real and serious matters.

Alzheimer's is now the most dreaded disease not only because of the devastating emotional effect it has on the Alzheimer's patient and the patient's family—but also because the cost for treating this incurable disease and caring for someone who is afflicted with it is enough to **bankrupt** any family.

It isn't just the high-profile, often terminal, diseases like cancer and AIDS that are getting expensive to treat. From the standpoint of our health care system, **Alzheimer's is the most costly disease** because it has become so *prevalent* and the cost per case has skyrocketed in recent years.

What are the chances that you or someone you care about will become afflicted with Alzheimer's? Here's the sobering news: One out of five people over 65—and 50% of people over age 85 are already afflicted with the disease (although some may not realize they have it).

What You Can Do to Prevent (or Even Reverse) the Disease

The most well-known risk factors for Alzheimer's are:

- Advanced age
- Low scores on tests of thinking skills
- Having the ApoE4 gene (which raises the genetic risks of developing Alzheimer's).

The risk factors most people don't know are the following:

> **Abstaining from alcohol** — That's right; NOT consuming alcohol may actually promote dementia. According to study findings presented at the Alzheimer's Association 2009 International Conference, having one or two alcoholic drinks per day may help prevent dementia in the elderly.

WARNING: Excessive alcohol use, however, may have the opposite effect and contribute to dementia.

> **Slowness of mind or movement** — This is indicative in approximately 50% of the cases of dementia that developed in a group of elderly people over a six-year period.

> **Being underweight**

> **Having a history of heart bypass surgery**

In addition, according to the results of a study published in the journal *Dementia and Geriatric Cognitive Disorders*, **high cholesterol levels** in midlife—even borderline high cholesterol—significantly increases the risk of Alzheimer's Disease 30 years later.

Unhealthy habits such as **smoking**, not doing physical activity, and not eating enough fruits and vegetables daily have also been linked to declining memory and thinking skills.

The good news is that now that you now know the risk factors, you can take steps to minimize your risk by simply doing the following:

1. Monitoring your weight (so as to avoid being underweight);

2. Keeping your cholesterol level in the healthy range;

3. Kicking the smoking habit;

4. Exercising more; and

5. Eating a sufficient amount of fruits and vegetables daily, and, of course,

6. Enjoying an alcoholic beverage each day.

Vitamin D: One of the
Best Ways to Reverse Asthma

Did You Know...
that one of the best asthma treatments is completely free?

More than twenty million adults in the United States have been diagnosed with asthma. Furthermore, nine million children suffer from asthma, making it the most prevalent chronic condition in children.

The most often prescribed asthma medications range from short-acting beta agonists (such as albuterol) to inhaled corticosteroids (such as Asmanex and Qvar) to leukotriene modifiers (such as Singulair and Zyflo) and to combination inhalers containing corticosteroids and long-acting beta agonists (such as Advair and Symbicort).

As is the case with most drugs, asthma medications come with their attendant side effects. Some side effects brought about by asthma drugs are *localized*—which means they appear in only one part of the body. Among these are reflex cough, bronchospasm, oral candidiasis (thrush) and dysphonia (hoarseness). Others are *systemic*, which means the effects are seen throughout the body. These include decreased bone density, poor growth, cataracts and glaucoma, adrenal gland suppression, Disseminated Varicella Infection (chickenpox that spreads to organs), and easy bruising.

One of the best ways to reverse asthma, however, does not involve the use of drugs. Severe asthma attacks have been closely linked to insufficient levels of Vitamin D in the body. In fact, a study published in the *Journal of Allergy and Clinical Immunology* confirms that **vitamin D insufficiency is linked to a 50% increase in the risk of severe asthma attacks**. If an asthma sufferer receives sufficient levels of Vitamin D, asthma attacks might be significantly minimized or even completely disappear.

The ideal source of Vitamin D is *sunlight*, which means the asthma solution is as close as the great outdoors, is completely free—and comes with no side effects (as long as you avoid excessive sun exposure).

For those who live in regions that don't get a lot of sunshine, or those who don't have time to receive the sun exposure necessary to soak up sufficient levels of Vitamin D, taking a high-quality Vitamin D supplement is advisable.

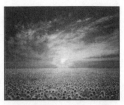

How much Vitamin D is necessary to achieve therapeutic effects, particularly in asthma cases? United States health agencies typically recommend 200 to 600 IUs of vitamin D per day. Unfortunately, the "healthy" vitamin D range recommended by these agencies is based on flawed and outdated guidelines, and is considered by most enlightened health practitioners to be grossly deficient.

Many health experts believe that the average person needs about 35 IUs of vitamin D per pound of body weight. Therefore, a person weighing 150 pounds needs 5,250 IUs, and a child weighing 60 pounds needs 2,100 IUs. Although this might seem like an extreme amount of vitamin D, to put it into the proper perspective, 1,000 IUs is only 25 micrograms or 0.025 milligrams. In some cases where severe vitamin D deficiency exists, the recommendations are even higher!

There are two types of vitamin D supplements; namely, vitamin D2 (ergocalciferol), which is found in plant sources, fortified foods and some supplements; and vitamin D3 (cholecalciferol), which comes from eggs, organ meats, animal fat, cod liver oil, and fish. Natural vitamin D3 (which is equivalent to the vitamin D3 produced from UV-B rays of the sun) is the type most often recommended for therapeutic reasons because it is far superior to synthetic vitamin D2, which has been shown to be toxic at higher doses.

Popular Japanese Breakfast Food Dissolves Blood Clots

Did You Know...

that there's Japanese food substance that dissolves blood clots better than any drug ... reduces blood pressure quickly ... and suppresses thickening of the arteries?

That substance is a sticky, cheese-like food called *natto*. It is produced by fermenting soybeans with the bacteria *Bacillus Subtilis*—one of the "good" bacteria that keeps the intestinal tract healthy and working properly. It has a nutty, salty flavor similar to Roquefort cheese. For over a thousand years, it has been a popular breakfast food in Japan, where it is eaten with rice. Now, it has been shown to 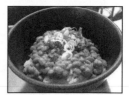 be a life-saving miracle treatment for cardiovascular disease—it has even been used to ward off heart disease, osteoporosis, cancer, and many other ailments.

In 1980, Dr. Hiroyuki Sumi, a chemist and researcher at the University of Chicago's Medical School, discovered the fibrinolytic (clot-busting) enzyme in natto called nattokinase. In one study, Dr. Sumi placed nattokinase on blood clots at body temperature **and the clots completely dissolved within eighteen hours**!

Further research has proven nattokinase effective in preventing heart attacks, strokes, cancer, bone fractures, and gastrointestinal problems. Every year, the Japanese consume 7.5 billion packets of natto; its consumption is believed to be the reason Japanese people live longer, have fewer heart attacks, and stronger bones than people in the United States.

Nattokinase is being hailed as the "miracle enzyme" because it has been scientifically proven to be one of the strongest defenses against heart disease—even when compared to pharmaceutical heart medications.

Nattokinase is especially **effective in dissolving fibrin**—a thread-like "web" that forms around injured red blood cells in order to stop bleeding, form a scab, and induce healing. While these are good things, if fibrin is not eliminated after it has done its job, it thickens and forms clots, which can lead to serious and sometimes fatal diseases such as heart disease, heart attack, and stroke.

The body naturally produces plasmin, which breaks up and dissolves fibrin, but with age, plasmin levels diminish and excess fibrin is left behind after an injury heals. Research shows that the nattokinase enzyme has four times the clot dissolving power of plasmin and supports heart health by:

• Stabilizing blood pressure

• Preventing the formation of unnecessary blood clots

• Dissolving excess fibrin and existing blood clots

• Boosting natural plasmin production and other clot-dissolving agents

One of the most beneficial effects of nattokinase is that it has an extremely powerful ability to disintegrate blood clots. Not only does it build your bones better than calcium, it's better and cheaper than any cholesterol-lowering drug (like Lipitor) to keep your heart healthy.

— Dr. Joseph Mercola, the publisher of a self-titled natural health newsletter and *New York Times* bestselling author

Dissolves More Clots than Drugs at a Fraction of the Cost!

Synthetic blood thinners are expensive, short acting, and have serious side effects. Investigative health reporters from *Medical Research Associates* confirmed that a single dose of pharmaceutical clot-dissolving drugs can cost as much as **$1,500**—and only actively dissolve clots for a few minutes to a half hour. Nattokinase, on the other hand, stays active in the body for eight to twelve hours and costs **less than $20.00.**

Nattokinase not only dissolves more clots faster, it also lowers cholesterol and blood pressure. Researchers from Oklahoma State University and Miyazaki Medical College tested nattokinase on twelve Japanese volunteers. The tests showed that the time it took to dissolve a blood clot dropped by 48% within 2 hours—and there was an **11% decrease in blood pressure after just 2 weeks**.

A study conducted in 2007 found that, "Among those who had high cholesterol (defined as greater than or equal to 220 mg/dl), eating one pack (30 grams) of natto every morning for four weeks **lowered their total cholesterol levels by an average of 8%**."

In addition to the enzyme nattokinase, natto also contains vitamin K2, which is naturally produced in the intestinal tract. As we age, production of this essential vitamin decreases. Vitamin K2 not only prevents hardening of the arteries and ensures proper blood clotting, it also helps the body "hang on" to calcium and deliver it directly to bones. Vitamin K has been found to be more effective than calcium in building stronger, denser bones for a **reduced risk of osteoporosis**.

A study published in the *Journal of Nutrition* in 2006, found that, "Women who ate more than four packets of natto per week (40 grams/packet) reduced bone mass loss at the top of their thigh bone by over 80% and in their lower arm by 60%."

Natto also contains **anti-tumor agents that fight cancer**. Its high levels of genistein (an isoflavone), phytoestrogen, and flavonoid compounds have anti-carcinogen properties that prevent chemotherapy and free radicals from damaging cells.

In addition to benefits that natto provides for heart, bone, and cellular health, it is also a *powerful probiotic*. Natto has been shown to reduce inflammation, alleviate gastrointestinal disorders (such as diarrhea and ulcers), and uro-genital conditions (such as urinary tract and yeast infections).

Natto has a pungent, "dirty sock" smell, a strong taste and a slimy texture. However, it can be purchased or prepared with other foods and flavors that make it more palatable. Many people find that taking a nattokinase supplement is pleasanter and more convenient—and it costs only $19.00. The recommended clot-dissolving supplement potency is 1,500 to 2,000 fibrin units (FUs) per capsule. Take one capsule a day as a dietary supplement, or as prescribed by your doctor or health practitioner.

Miracle Compound Speeds Healing

Did You Know...

that there is a "miracle" compound that has the power to relieve pain, diminish swelling, reduce inflammation, encourage healing, restore normal cell function and even eliminate scar tissue?

Dimethyl sulfoxide (DMSO), a simple by-product of the wood industry, is the compound that even doctors are calling a "wonderful medical miracle."

It was first synthesized by Russian scientist Alexander Saytzeff in 1866. But it wasn't until after World War II that chemists began to discover that DMSO could *dissolve almost anything* and *carry any dissolved substances along with it*. For this reason, it has long been used as an industrial solvent.

DMSOs medicinal properties came to light in 1961 when Dr. Stanley Jacob, head of the organ transplant program at Oregon Health Sciences University picked up a bottle of the colorless liquid in his search for a preservative for organs. During his investigation of DMSOs, he discovered that it had the ability to **penetrate the skin quickly and deeply**—without damaging the skin.

Indeed, it has been observed that if someone were to apply a small amount of the DMSO liquid on the sole of their foot, it would penetrate through the skin and travel through the body at such extreme speed that the person would "taste" the DMSO almost instantly.

DMSO is said to be more "liquid" than water and has been shown to penetrate areas in the body that nothing else can reach as fast. Because it moves rapidly through cell membranes, it has been called "water's alter ego." It changes the water structure within the cell, increases cellular permeability, and accelerates the living processes of the cell thereby allowing healing to occur at unprecedented speed.

DMSO Speeds All Healing — Doubling or Tripling Healing Response Times

DMSO has been shown to relieve pain and swelling, relax muscles, relieve arthritis, improve blood supply and slow the growth of bacteria.

In an article entitled *"DMSO As a Solvent,"* Dr. Ron Kennedy reports: It relieves the pain of sprains and even of broken bones. It enhances the effectiveness of other pharmacological agents. **If you apply DMSO to a bruise, the bruise dissolves and disappears in a matter of minutes!** If you apply it to the jaw after wisdom tooth removal, *all pain and swelling is prevented!* The pain of **acute gout** can be handled with the application of 5 cc of seventy percent DMSO in water four times each day. Application to a **fever blister** results in rapid resolution of this problem. DMSO also relieves the pain of minor burns and if applied soon after the burn happens, will decrease the tissue damage suffered. DMSO speeds all healing, approximately doubling or tripling all healing responses.

In addition to providing great relief for sufferers of osteoarthritis, rheumatoid arthritis, burns, sprains, back and neck problems, DMSO also delivers antibacterial, antiviral and antifungal effects.

For example:

> ➤ If administered intravenously within 90 minutes of a stroke, it prevents permanent damage to the central nervous system.

> ➤ When applied topically, repeatedly, **it flattens a raised keloid scar**. It also prevents the contracture of scar tissue that accompanies burns.

> ➤ It protects against the tissue damage induced by radiation.

> ➤ It prevents tissue damage ordinarily caused by freezing conditions.

> ➤ It minimizes the swelling of the brain and spinal cord following traumatic injury.

In 1972, the painkilling ability of DMSO attracted media attention when Dr. Jacob administered it to Governor George Wallace. Wallace had been wounded in an assassination attempt while campaigning for the Democratic nomination for president. As a result, he was wheelchair-bound and afflicted with pain. His pain reportedly disappeared after applying DMSO daily over the affected area.

DMSO attained even more widespread recognition when the popular television program *60 Minutes* aired a presentation entitled "The Riddle of DMSO" on March 23, 1980, and again on July 6 of that same year. The show reached the homes of 70 million viewers, and as a result, Dr. Jacob's office was swamped with thousands of phone calls from pain victims clamoring for the miracle painkiller called DMSO. The phones of other physicians who were known to prescribe DMSO also rang continuously for several days following the broadcast of *60 Minutes*.

DMSO has been used most widely as a topical analgesic, in a solution consisting of 70% DMSO and 30% water. Laboratory studies show that DMSO cuts pain by blocking peripheral nerve C fibers. Relief from the pain of burns, cuts, and sprains has been reported to be almost immediate and to last up to six hours.

DMSO is also widely used in sports medicine. Professional sports organizations, in particular, use it to help athletes recover from injury and back onto the playing field rapidly.

Dr. Jacob said at a hearing of the U.S. Senate Subcommittee on Health in 1980:

> DMSO is one of the few agents in which **effectiveness can be demonstrated before the eyes of the observers** .... If we have patients appear before the Committee with edematous sprained ankles, the application of DMSO would be followed by objective diminution of swelling *within an hour*. No other therapeutic modality will do this.

Despite overwhelming evidence pointing to DMSO's therapeutic benefits, and in spite of the fact that DMSO is known to be safer than aspirin, the Food and Drug Administration (FDA) refuses to approve the use or prescription of DMSO for anything other than the treatment of an obscure bladder condition called interstitial cystitis.

Eight states have effectively bypassed the authority of the FDA because their respective state legislatures have legalized the prescribing of DMSO. These states are Florida, Louisiana, Montana, Nevada, Oklahoma, Oregon, Texas and Washington. In these states, doctors who are experienced with DMSO often use intravenous drips to treat the symptoms of cancer, atherosclerosis, Parkinson's disease, multiple sclerosis and arthritis.

Legally, DMSO is sold commercially only as a solvent. However, that hasn't stopped osteoarthritis and rheumatoid arthritis sufferers from using it with regularity, often at the recommendation of fellow arthritis sufferers.

WARNING: "Only medical grade—never industrial grade—should be used on the human body," insists Dr. Ron Kennedy. That's because the industrial grade DMSO contains acetone and acid contaminants.

Medical grade DMSO is available from Terra Pharmaceuticals, in Buena Park, California. Distributors, such as Rimso and Domoso, obtain it from this source and put their private label on it. DMSO is available at health food stores and from online retailers.

Zap Viruses and
Harmful Bacteria Disappear!

Did You Know...

that there's a way to make viruses and harmful bacteria disappear in three minutes?

In 1995, Dr. Hulda Clark, a naturopath and physiologist, presented fascinating information in her book, *The Cure for All Diseases*, about a hand-held electronic device that anyone can build at home at a cost of $20 to $30. The battery-operated device, which Dr. Clark developed, was called *The Zapper*—and she used it to cure a wide variety of ailments and diseases, including cancer.

The Zapper essentially **electrocutes pathogens** using a positive offset 30 KHz square wave frequency. It imparts a very small electric current through the body when the user holds two copper electrodes with an output voltage of about five volts apiece. The current is only a couple of miliamperes, and The Zapper pulses the current, which has the effect of reducing the skin's natural resistance to electrical current.

The Zapper used by Dr. Clark in her clinic **causes viruses and bacteria to disappear within three minutes**. Tapeworm stages and roundworms are eradicated in five minutes, and mites are gone in seven minutes. However, "zapping" does not destroy good bacteria. Although fast results occur within three to seven minutes, the treatment protocol calls for holding the electrodes for twenty to thirty minutes, three times a day, with seven-minute intervals between zaps.

When The Zapper pulses the current, it introduces negative electrons through the skin and into the body's living tissue. Since all parasites and diseased tissues are positively charged (i.e., they are composed of atoms or groups of atoms that have a shortage of electrons), introducing negative electrons reverses *their polarity*, killing the parasites and helping to heal the diseased tissue. The Zapper has also been shown to inactivate toxins in the body. In her book, *The Cure for All Diseases*, Dr. Clark provides complete instructions on how to build a zapper.

Some people have found Dr. Clark's Zapper a bit cumbersome to use because you have to hold the copper electrodes in both hands, and sit in that position through the entire treatment. Other natural health practitioners have since developed devices (emulating Dr. Clark's original Zapper) that are more convenient to use.

Perhaps the most popular of these derivative devices is the one developed by Don Croft, who created a version of the zapper in a 2" x 3" plastic box which employs two copper pennies positioned an inch apart on top of the unit as electrodes.

Don Croft's zapper, which he calls *The Terminator*, is easy to use because it can be attached to the arm with an elastic band—the electrodes (copper pennies) touch the skin. Because of its size and the way it is attached to the arm, it offers the added convenience of allowing the user to move around freely while "zapping." It works in exactly the same way as The Zapper, but it also uses the power of orgonite. There are numerous anecdotal reports of The Terminators ability to "cure" a range of illnesses including **cancer, lupus, migraines, herpes, depression, colitis, ulcers**, and a **wide variety of other ailments**.

Ready-made zappers like Don Croft's Terminator are available on the Internet.

WARNING: Pregnant women and people with pacemakers are advised not to use zappers since the effects on them are not as yet known.

As with any unconventional healing modality that mainstream medicine brands "questionable," zappers have had their share of critics and naysayers. Some have said they are akin to *snake oil*, and Hulda Clark has been called a *quack*. But then again, so have many doctors who have dared to present healing concepts that are not endorsed by the medical establishment or Big Pharma. Dr. Clark has been the subject of many attacks by professional adversaries, and has been in legal battles which were eventually dismissed by courts.

There is definitely solid science behind Dr. Clark's zapper technology —whether organized medicine acknowledges it as valid or not. You don't have to fully understand how a zapper works in order to benefit from it. The only way to know for certain is to suspend your judgment long enough to try it.

I have been using Don Croft's zapper with great results since 2003. It's available at www.worldwithoutparasites.com. When you quickly cure yourself of acute or chronic illness with a zapper, it's an empowering feeling.

WARNING: Don't Take Antioxidants Until You Read This!

Did You Know...

that high doses of antioxidant supplements — such as beta carotene, Vitamin A, Vitamin E, ascorbic acid (Vitamin C) and selenium—do not reduce the risk of disease, can be poisonous, and may even increase the risk of death?

As long ago as the 1950s, antioxidants became known as miracle supplements because they reportedly promoted good health and prevented a host of diseases, including cancer and age-related diseases. According to some estimates, approximately 50% of the adult population in the U.S. take antioxidants on a daily basis for this reason.

This is a wake-up call: every long-term study involving antioxidant supplementation provides proof that people get sicker—not healthier—when they take antioxidants. In fact, beta carotene, vitamin A, and vitamin E, taken individually or in combination with other antioxidant supplements, are associated with increased all-cause mortality.[6] (385 publications).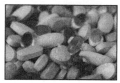

In case you were wondering, this information is not just "more propaganda"from the medical and pharmaceutical industries to prevent people from using natural therapies, or to deceive people into thinking that drugs are the only solution to disease.

Here are the facts: over the last several decades, supplement manufacturers (and even health practitioners) have urged people to take large amounts of antioxidants such as Vitamin C and Vitamin E because scientists had observed that people whose diets were rich in fruits and vegetables had a lower incidence of heart disease, diabetes, dementia, stroke and certain types of cancer. They formed the hypothesis that since fruits and vegetables are a rich source of antioxidants (which neutralize free radicals in the body), then taking antioxidant supplements would have the same effect.

That hypothesis has been proven wrong. Here's why: fruits and vegetables produce antioxidants for a good reason—to protect themselves from

---

[6] *The Journal of the American Medical Association* report on a study based on 68 randomized trials with 232,606 participants (385 publications).

oxidative stress. Without antioxidants, oxygen would destroy food by combining with elements and essentially burning them up—the result, vitamin destruction (or decay) occurs.

Dietary antioxidants like beta carotene, vitamin A, and vitamin E, have virtually no nutritional benefit. Antioxidants such as ascorbic acid and tocopherols, for instance, are not essential nutrients—and should not even be called vitamins at all.

While antioxidants serve their purpose *within* a fruit or vegetable, isolated antioxidants consumed by humans tend to disrupt normal oxidative reactions in the cell, and, for this reason, it is dangerous to consume them (except in the minute amounts ingested from food).

If you want to stave off disease and premature aging, there is no substitute for eating fruits and vegetables that are rich in antioxidants instead of antioxidant supplements.

WARNING: Popular Arthritis Medication Accelerates Cartilage Breakdown

Did You Know...

that a supposedly "safe" and popular arthritis pill actually accelerates cartilage breakdown? Thousands of innocent victims take this pill daily without knowing the real risks.

Non-steroidal anti-inflammatory drugs (usually abbreviated to NSAIDs), are drugs with analgesic (pain-reducing) and antipyretic (fever-reducing) effects. They are among the most widely used drugs throughout the developed world.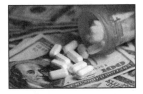

According to a report published in *Clinical Cornerstone,*[7] NSAIDs annually account for 70 million prescriptions and 30 billion over-the-counter (OTC) medications sold in the United States alone. They are usually indicated for the treatment of acute or chronic conditions where pain and inflammation are present—and that includes *arthritis*.

---

[7]Green, Gary, MD, "Understanding NSAIDs: From aspirin to COX-2" *Clinical Cornerstone*, 3:50-59, 2001

Most people are not aware of the well-established fact that traditional NSAIDs **accelerate cartilage destruction and inhibit cartilage formation.** Many studies have confirmed this, and it has been known for decades. It's quite ironic that the very same drugs indicated for the *symptomatic relief* of arthritis actually contribute to its progression!

The Encyclopedia of Medical Breakthroughs and Forbidden Treatments states:

In 1979, physicians in Norway made x-ray evaluations of the hips of 58 patients taking Indicin® (indomethacin). Patients taking the NSAID experienced significantly more rapid destruction of the hip than the control group taking no NSAIDs. Studies with aspirin and other NSAIDs have repeated these results.[8]

Some of the most popular NSAIDs are **ibuprofen** (Advil and Motrin), naproxen sodium (*Aleve*), ketoprofen (*Orudis KT*) as well as **aspirin**. Therefore, when you take these pain medications to relieve headaches, migraines, menstrual pain, postoperative pain, metastatic bone pain or any kind of pain—or to bring a fever down—you are actually accelerating cartilage breakdown.

Cartilage breakdown is not the only adverse effect of NSAID use, however. The two main adverse drug reactions (ADRs) associated with NSAIDs relate to gastrointestinal (GI) effects and renal effects. In addition, the investigative medical journalists at Medical Research Associates report that researchers at the University of Newcastle in Australia have discovered that NSAID use is a **significant contributor to congestive heart failure** (CHF). CHF is failure of the heart muscle including its ability to maintain adequate blood circulation throughout the body or to pump out the venous blood as it returns to the heart.

---

[8] Roningen, H., et al. "Indomethacin treatment in osteoporosis of the hip joint." *Acta Orthopdica Scandanavica*, 50:168-174, 1979; Newman, N.M., et al. "Acetabular bone destruction related to nonsteroidal anti-inflammatory drugs." *Lancet*, ii:11-13, 1985; Solomon, I. "Drug-induced arthropathy and necrosis of the femoral head." Journal of Bone and Joint Surgery, 55B:246-251, 1973

How to Stop Sugar Cravings

Did You Know...

that you can stop sugar cravings with an adequate amount of two trace minerals?

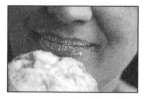

If you frequently crave candy bars, doughnuts, cake, or other sugary foods—and you *thought* your cravings were just something you were born with, or a condition to which you were naturally or *genetically predisposed*, there is hard scientific evidence that suggests otherwise.

There is a condition called **pica**, which triggers the craving for sweets —and it is caused by **mineral deficiencies**.

An example of pica in the animal world is seen in young calves that are raised for veal. These calves are deficient in iron. They are put into cages soon after birth and purposely fed a diet that is iron-poor so that they grow to be anemic. Anemic calves produce the pale, tender meat that makes veal desirable to food enthusiasts. The iron-starved calves have been known to seek, lick and chew on the iron nails of their cages in an effort to satisfy their hunger for iron. (We do not support such cruelty to animals; we present this example merely to illustrate the effect of pica in animals.)

In humans, an extreme example of pica is seen in pregnant women, who often crave things like ice cream or pickles, and especially non-food items like laundry starch, clay or dirt. These cravings occur because the fetus absorbs many of the minerals from the woman's body and the woman is looking for something that will satisfy her mineral deficiency.

Pica has become a common condition primarily because our de-mineralized soils yield mineral-poor produce. In addition, food processing robs food of important nutrients, which also contributes to the prevalence of pica—especially among people who do not consume balanced diets—dieters, vegetarians, meat eaters, teenagers, children and seniors.

When you crave sweets, eating highly sweetened food such as doughnuts and chocolates may temporarily satisfy your sugar craving, but it does very little to alleviate the mineral deficiency, which is the underlying cause of the cravings. Studies show that sugar cravings are linked to a deficiency in the trace minerals, **chromium** and **vanadium**. It is scientifically proven that both chromium and vanadium help in normalizing blood sugar. Both trace minerals have been shown to be essential for normal glucose metabolism. This is why they have also been used to prevent and cure diabetes (high blood sugar) and hypoglycemia (low blood sugar).

A chromium deficiency has been shown to not only cause cravings for sugars or starches, but also contribute to poor muscle tone, which makes weight loss even more difficult. To help curb sugar cravings, many health practitioners prescribe a daily intake of both chromium and vanadium, preferably taken in ionic/water soluble form for maximum absorption. Many health food stores carry ionic minerals. You can also type the keyword "ionic minerals" onto any search engine to find online retailers, such as the Water Oz company, which manufactures high quality chromium and vanadium formulations.

Chocolate cravings, in particular, are curbed by magnesium supplementation. Magnesium is also contained in commercially available ionic/water soluble mineral formulations.

Whey Protein: The Best Protein Source for Burning Body Fat

Did You Know...
that whey protein can turn your body into a fat-burning furnace?

Whey is a milk-based protein which is a by-product of cheese production. It has the highest biological value among all proteins. This means that it has a higher amino acid content, and is the most easily absorbed by the body compared to other rich sources of protein, including milk, soy and egg whites.

Everyone knows that in order to attain an attractive, *well-defined*, firm and **youthful body**, one needs... protein, protein and more protein! When it comes to shaping your body, nothing is more important than building lean muscle. And when it comes to building muscle, nothing is more important than getting the right amount of protein. Here's why:

Protein contains four calories per gram, but when it's being digested, it burns six calories per gram. Therefore, whereas both carbohydrates and fat burn calories equivalent to their respective caloric values, *protein burns 50% more calories.* 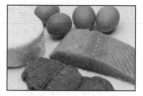 A diet rich in protein can also **raise your resting metabolic rate by as much as 68%**. Simply said, just by eating protein, you immediately speed up your metabolic furnace, thereby enabling your body to increase lean muscle mass and **accelerate the fat-burning process**.

Whey protein is arguably the best protein source for building lean muscles. Many people have found that consuming a good whey protein supplement in addition to the protein they derive from meat and fish, is the ideal way to fortify their body with extra protein—especially because the body assimilates whey protein better than hard-to-digest animal flesh. Furthermore, *it doesn't have the saturated fats* that beef and other animal proteins have.

Whey also has medicinal properties, and has been proven to **prevent cancer** in animals. It has been shown to provide an extra boost to the immune system by increasing glutathione (GSH) levels in cancer patients, or patients with the Human Immunodeficiency Virus (HIV), because whey protein is rich in the amino acid cysteine.

Whey protein powder is widely used by athletes and body builders, who consume 60 grams or more per day to maintain their muscle mass. That level of whey protein intake, however, is excessive for the average individual. If you have a sedentary, non-athletic lifestyle, and you wish to use whey to support your weight loss goals, many people find that 20 to 40 grams a day is sufficient. For medicinal purposes, 40 to 80 grams has been shown to be ideal.

An often overlooked use of whey protein is help prevent bone loss and limit muscle loss over time—something especially useful for **senior citizens**. Many nutritionists believe that whey protein should be part of every senior citizen's diet.

Whey protein powder is widely available at health food stores (such as Whole Foods), supplement stores (such as Vitamin Shoppe), and from countless online retailers.

Always choose the *non-denatured type* of whey protein because the process of denaturation breaks down the natural protein structures and minimizes their biological activity. Select a whey protein manufacturer that does not expose the whey to high temperatures (which negatively affects protein quality), and one that carefully does everything to preserve the vital whey protein fractions, such as the health-promoting immune-globulins, glycomacropeptides, lactoferrin, etc. One such product is Designer Whey Protein manufactured by Next Proteins.

WARNING: If you have milk allergies, you should try a small amount of whey protein initially to make sure you can tolerate the specific whey product you're using. As with all supplementation, consult your medical practitioner for advice.

A "Broom for the Stomach": Sweep Away 25% of the Calories You Eat

Did You Know...
that a Japanese potato called *konnyaku* can flush 25% of the calories you eat out of your body?

Konnyaku is a traditional Japanese food made from the *corm* (the short, thick food-storing underground stem) of the konnyaku potato or konjac plant (Amorphophallus konjac), also known as the Devil's Tongue plant. Konnyaku potatoes are cultivated for food only in Japan, but it grows wild in many warm 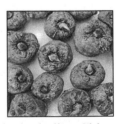 subtropical to tropical areas in eastern and southern Asia, including China and Indonesia.

This fat-free, virtually zero-calorie food, which has been used as an ingredient in Japanese dishes for over 2,000 years, consists of 97% water and 3% glucomannan, a viscous fiber. It also contains traces of protein, starch and minerals like calcium.

Glucomannan is an amazingly dense, high fiber substance that has the ability to **expand to 200 times its size** upon entering the digestive tract. It envelops calories, carbohydrates and fats in fiber. Therefore, as food passes through your digestive system, the body reacts to them as if they were fiber, and flushes them out of your body, along with any toxins in your digestive tract. It's no wonder the Japanese call it a "broom for the stomach."

For weight management purposes, many people use konjac glucomannan in the following forms:

➤ **Konjac Glucomannan Powder**: There are several ways to use the powder form:

- ✓ Three times daily—before each meal, stir one level teaspoon of the powder (about 4 grams) briskly in one cup of water, and drink it before it begins to gel.
- ✓ Sprinkle the powder on your food to block calories

When swallowed, the glucomannan expands into a fibrous gel and traps food particles. It also **creates a feeling of fullness**; as a result you eat less. This allows you to maintain weight without experiencing the side effects that accompany most fat blockers.

➤ **Konnyaku Noodles**: Konnyaku formed into noodles called *shirataki*, which means "white waterfall." Shirataki noodles are translucent, gelatinous, wheat- and gluten-free, and are available in most Asian markets. These noodles should not be confused with the shirataki noodles sold in Whole Foods Markets, which are *made of tofu*, not pure konjac or konnyaku. Shirataki noodles have very little flavor of their own, and because they consist of 97% water, they readily absorb the dominant flavor of any soup or dish in which they are cooked. You can combine shirataki noodles with all kinds of flavorful ingredients to create virtually zero-calorie bulk to fill up those hungry spaces in your belly.

And because these noodles contain **zero net carbohydrates** and **zero calories**, they make for a "guiltless pasta" indulgence. Simply toss or stir-fry the noodles with teriyaki sauce, vinegar, soy sauce, hot salsa, your favorite pasta sauce or ingredients like pepper, onion, or garlic to make a quick meal.

If there are no nearby Asian markets, you can purchase these products from a number of online retailers. Simply type the following keywords onto any search engine: "konjac glucomannan powder" or "konnyaku noodles where to buy" or visit KonjacFoods.com.

Rub Your Stomach Away
in Just Two Minutes a Day

Did You Know...

that you can rub your stomach away effortlessly using nothing but your hand—for only 2 minutes a day?

This may sound hard to believe, but Dr. Stephen Chang, an M.D. and Ph.D. who is trained in both Western and Chinese medicine, states that this simple two-minute internal exercise, which has been handed down from ancient Chinese sages, has been used successfully as a self-healing mechanism for over 6,000 years.

Whatever you do, don't confuse this **internal exercise** with the *external exercises* that are popular in the West, such as sit-ups, crunches and other movements that only firm up the underlying stomach muscles, but do nothing to melt the fat surrounding those muscles,.

According to Dr. Chang, losing weight is a simple matter of increasing the efficiency of the digestive system. If you've ever wondered why you fail to shed pounds even when you reduce the amount of food you eat and/or your caloric intake—the reason is because your digestive and eliminatory systems are not functioning efficiently.

The following two-minute exercise works like a gentle colonic irrigation and helps **speed up a sluggish digestive system** (which usually carries at least five pounds of fecal matter within it, and eliminating this useless sludge has the effect of **burning off excess fat**. The exercise effectively metabolizes the fatty tissues around the stomach and intestines, and flushes them out of your body through blood, sweat, urine, and feces.

Here's how to do the stomach-rubbing exercise:

1. Lie flat on your back on your bed or on the floor. Take your top off or pull it up so that your abdominal area is bare.

2. Rub your hands together vigorously for about fifteen seconds, or until they feel hot.

3. Place one of your hands directly on your belly button and begin to rub making small circles around your belly button.

Gradually make the circles larger. Use a fairly firm but comfortable pressure and rub at a slow, even pace, approximately one circle per second.

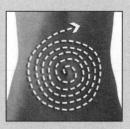

4. Concentrate on the heat building up in, around and throughout your stomach.

5. Do about 40 to 50 circles, or for approximately two minutes or more.

Note: It is important to keep the abdominal area warm while doing the exercise, especially during winter months when even heated indoor air tends to be cool.

For best results, do this routine twice a day for two minutes—first thing in the morning (before breakfast) and just before you go to bed. Most people see noticeable results within one week of consistent practice.

According to traditional Chinese medicine, the stomach is the center of energy. For this reason, this stomach massage actually accomplishes more than just melting away adipose tissue (fat).

It also helps:

✓ Stimulate the abdominal organs

✓ Speed up slow digestion and remedy constipation

✓ Increase blood circulation in the abdominal area

✓ Heal indigestion, nausea, diarrhea, vomiting and the adverse effects of overeating

WARNING: Do not do the stomach massage exercise immediately after a heavy meal. Neither is it recommended for women who are pregnant, or have inflammation of the uterus, bladder, ovaries or fallopian tubes or individuals with the following conditions: hypertension; stones in the gall bladder, kidneys or bladder; general, femoral, inguinal and umbilical hernia; bleeding of the stomach, lungs or brain; or ulcers of the intestines or stomach.

PART TWO

What You Can Do...

News You Can Use: Noteworthy Article Contributions from UHR's Partners

Prologue: Shocking Confessions of a Drug Company Insider

This story seems to be ripped from the headlines—or maybe a movie about a big *conspiracy or a cover-up of foul play*—just like the Oscar award-winning *"The Insider."*

But it is 100% true.

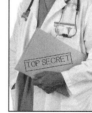

In 2003, a top executive of the pharmaceutical giant GlaxoSmithKline—worldwide vice president of genetics —confessed that **"The vast majority of drugs—more than 90%—only work in 30 or 50% of the people."**

That means that *most prescription drugs DON'T work on most of the people who take them!*

Dr. Allen Roses is the pharmaceutical industry insider who made this **shocking confession**. Although it's been an open secret in the pharmaceutical industry that most of the drugs it produces are ineffective in most patients, this is the first time that a high-ranking pharmaceutical executive has gone public.

Some industry analysts said that the confession of Dr. Roses is reminiscent of the famous words uttered by Gerald Ratner, a British retail magnate in 1991, who said that his High Street shops were successful because they sold "total crap."

But it's one thing for a company to sell *worthless* products and another to sell worthless **products that actually kill** instead of heal.

FACT: In the United States, the odds of being killed by conventional medicine are almost **20 times (2,000%) greater than being killed in an automobile accident** and almost **30 times (3,000%) greater than being killed by a gun**.

111

It's no wonder that the majority of doctors are *frustrated*. They entered the medical profession wanting to cure people—but the only tools that medical school training provides them for treating patients are **drugs** and **surgery**.

Doctors have been thrust headlong into a marketing culture that relies on selling as many drugs as possible to the widest number of patients. It's a culture that has made Big Pharma the most profitable industry in the world—even though most of its drugs are useless, at best—and possibly harmful or deadly for many patients.

Dr. Roses, an academic geneticist from Duke University in North Carolina, further states: "Drugs for Alzheimer's disease work in *fewer than one in three patients*, whereas those for cancer are only *effective in a quarter of patients*. Drugs for migraines, for osteoporosis, and arthritis work in *about half the patients*."

The growing sentiment among doctors is that they want to offer their patients more treatment choices for curing disease than the medical system offers. One member of that growing number of doctors is Dr. Paul Beals, who stated:

> I want to do more for my patients than what's offered by the pharmaceutical industry because I realized earlier on that **modern medicine has become, unfortunately, more of a big business than a healing science.**"
>
> – Paul Beals, M.D., C.C.N., Georgetown University School of Medicine (Course Instructor 1996-2004: *Introduction to Complementary and Alternative Medicine*)

When Doctors Don't Know the Cure, This is What They Turn To

Some time ago, Dr. Beals focused his medical practice on holistic nutrition and complementary medicine. He set up a holistic program for cancer, heart disease, diabetes, stroke, liver disease, and other diseases. His challenge, however, was finding alternative resources for treating these diseases because conventional medicine offered only drugs and surgery.

He stumbled upon a book titled *The Encyclopedia of Medical Breakthroughs and Forbidden Treatments* that contained **all the cures** he was looking for. Interestingly, the book was *written for the layperson*—the general public—not medical professionals. And yet Beals was impressed to discover that every alternative treatment and healing breakthrough presented in the book was **thoroughly researched**, meticulously fact-checked and verified for its effectiveness. It was fully footnoted with citations from **peer-reviewed, published medical research** and **scientific studies**. He now regards the book as the gold standard, the "bible for alternative medicine," and believes **"It should be in everybody's home and in every doctor's office."**

Dr. Beals is not alone in his high regard for the book. Countless enlightened doctors from around the world are avid fans and use the treatments presented in the book when they or their family members are stricken with diseases or health problems.

Dr. Russell Simmons thinks that everyone needs this book of medical breakthroughs and "forbidden treatments" in order to take control of their own health. Dr. Simmons is a medical doctor who sits on the faculty at Ohio State University, where he's an Associate Professor of Ophthalmology. He's also the Chairman of the Alternative Medicine Committee of the Columbus Medical Association.

Dr. Simmons's wife developed cancer six years ago, and underwent surgery which put her cancer in temporary remission. A year ago, her cancer returned. This time, instead of turning to conventional cancer therapy, Simmons and his wife turned to the discoveries presented in the book to help p*revent further surgery and further progression of the disease.*

A doctor friend of Dr. Simmons, whose practice is based in Hawaii, started developing **cataracts**. A chapter of the book revealed a discovery about some little-known eye drops, which he began administering to himself; he noticed significant improvement in his vision. He continues to take the drops to this day.

The Encyclopedia of Medical Breakthroughs and Forbidden Treatments contains dozens of cures for the most prevalent diseases that plague mankind, such as:

> ➤ **A $200 "Cure" for AIDS / HIV**: A patented low-voltage device that stops the AIDS virus dead in its tracks. This inexpensive "in-home" device costs only $200, and is safe for home use.

> **Two Common Household Items that "Cure" Cancer**: A Nobel Prize nominee came up with a simple protocol for cancer treatment and prevention based on the use of small amounts of two inexpensive food substances combined in specific proportions.

Numerous independent clinical studies prove that these two food items provide a powerful and effective means of treating even the most advanced cancers. This method was shown to have a 90% success rate in saving terminal cancer patients from certain death.

> **An Infra-Red Helmet with a 90% Success Rate in Halting the Progression of Alzheimer's Disease**: There's a space-age helmet that uses new "light beam" technology to reverse Alzheimer's in as little as 30 days when used for ten minutes a day!

> **An Extremely Potent Anti-Inflammatory Breakthrough Does Wonders for Arthritis Sufferers**: Over three decades of painstaking research has led to the development of an anti-inflammation remedy that reduces swollen joints by 79%! The anti-arthritic marine lipids derived from a New Zealand mollusk have been tested extensively at the University of Queensland in Australia - and the results are quite dramatic!

> **An Herb that Virtually Eradicates Heart Disease**: There's an herb that has been used overseas to treat over 15,000 cardiac patients over a twenty-year period—and there have been no recurrences of the disease.

Dr. Roth Andersen, a doctor of naturopathic medicine and chiropractic physician, was constantly looking for ways to identify the root cause(s) of his patients' problems. He devoted many years of study looking for answers to the diverse health problems of his patients. He, too, found the answers he was looking for in *The Encyclopedia of Medical Breakthroughs and Forbidden Treatments*, which has been praised by laypeople and doctors alike.

This book goes far beyond anything that I've ever used," said Dr. Andersen. It's absolutely one of a kind ... It's so complete, so precise, so easy to use." He particularly appreciates how simple it is for anyone to look up a disease in the index, then flip to the page(s) of the book that features the disease—and find treatments, procedures, healing modalities, and supplements that are not only effective, but also **inexpensive, non-invasive,** and **free of side effects**.

This book is something that every alternative physician ... and ultimately every regular physician, and **every patient is going to want in their home or office** so that they can get the most benefit and the answers that are necessary to get their health condition handled.

Books offering miracle cures for practically every disease are available everywhere. But often, they present content that is erroneous, inaccurate, poorly researched—and *unsubstantiated* by science. It's no wonder that doctors and scientists ridicule such "cures" as nothing more than folklore or kitchen table wisdom.

Go to: http://undergroundhealthreporter.com/encymedical for more information about real cures for virtually every disease, and read David Allen's special report titled *Open the Door to a New World of Healing Options*.

Chapter 9 - Aging Well:
How to Look and Feel Your Best

One of the Most Important Things
You Can Do to Live Longer

Have you ever wondered why some people who eat a balanced and wholesome diet, exercise regularly, and live a healthy lifestyle sometimes age rapidly and prematurely while others who drink, smoke, eat junk food and live unhealthy lifestyles sometimes look youthful and **live to a ripe old age** without many health problems?

The reason may well lie in the levels of an enzyme that exists in the body known as Superoxide Dismutase.

Levels of Superoxide Dismutase (SOD) vary by as much as 50% among individuals, which may explain why some people age quickly and others live happy, healthy, relatively problem-free lives well into their 90s, or even 100 and beyond.

What is SOD—and why is it such a **critical measure of longevity**, seemingly outweighing other aging factors like diet, exercise, and, even, smoking?

Fruit Flies to Live Twice As Long with SOD!

Superoxide Dismutase (SOD) is a class of enzymes that repairs cells and reduces the cellular damage caused by the most common free radical in the body called superoxide. SOD acts as a catalyst which causes the dismutation—a process of simultaneous oxidation and reduction—of superoxide into *oxygen* and *hydrogen peroxide*. As a result, it provides the cells with an important antioxidant defense—one that is **3,500 times more powerful than Vitamin C**.

In addition, SOD acts as an anti-inflammatory, **neutralizing the free radicals that can lead to wrinkles** and precancerous cell changes.

Researchers have been studying the potential of superoxide dismutase as an **anti-aging treatment**, since it was discovered that SOD levels drop as we age—the same time that free radical levels increase.

A small number of little-known aging studies found that animals that produce the highest levels of SOD have the longest life spans. When the researchers genetically engineered fruit flies to produce double the amount of this super enzyme, **the fruit flies lived twice as long**!

Based on this, you might be inclined to run to the nearest health food store to buy a Superoxide Dismutase supplement. But there's actually much more to it than that: SOD is such a *fragile* molecule, and, for that reason, until recently, it was impossible for it to get through your digestive system without being destroyed. Ongoing research has shown that:

✓ Free SOD is destroyed in the stomach.

✓ Oral supplementation of free SOD does not increase tissue SOD activity.

✓ A small percentage of SOD can be placed in the intestinal tract but cannot get past the gastrointestinal (GI) barrier.

Patented Technology Allows SOD to Be Efficiently Absorbed

Not long ago, scientists discovered a way to wrap SOD in a protective coating, which allows it to be sent through your digestive tract without being damaged. Once the SOD gets past your stomach, it's efficiently absorbed—with all its potency intact—by your small intestine.

This remarkable technology has been patented (U.S. Patent 6 04 5809) and represents an exciting breakthrough in the field of anti-aging. For the first time in medical history, you now have a way to get more SOD into your body and actually increase your health span. Thus far, **this new kind of SOD is the only way to boost your body's level of SOD**.

Dr. Al Sears, a leading expert on anti-aging, states: "Your genetics are not written in stone. You have more control over your aging process than you think." Although he continues to emphasize that it's still important to eat a healthy diet and exercise regularly, he believes that increasing your level of SOD has a powerful impact on how long you live, even if you have other risk factors.

How SOD Protects Your DNA

SOD makes every cell in your body more resilient and able to fight off attacks better from the outside. No other antioxidant—not carotenoids, nor flavonoids, nor Vitamins A, C and E, nor CoQ10, and not even Glutathione Peroxidase and Catalase come close to the power of SOD.

SOD safeguards your DNA, the blueprint your body uses to build every organ, tissue and cell in your body. In a randomized, placebo-controlled study, researchers exposed two groups of people to high-pressure oxygen. The result was *oxidation*, 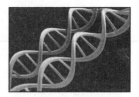 which is similar to what happens when you slice an apple and leave it exposed to the air for an hour. The oxygen causes the apple to turn brown and eventually spoil. In the body, oxidation affects the cellular membranes and their DNA, which wears out the cells, and eventually causes aging.

In the study, the control group's delicate strands of DNA broke. But the cellular membranes of the group taking the new SOD remained virtually intact and there was *no breakage in the DNA strands*.

SOD supports your immune system and safeguards your DNA in a way that **fights off the devastating forces of aging**. Therefore, one of the most important things you can do to live longer and enjoy better health as you age is to raise your levels of SOD.

Four Crucial Steps You Must Take Once Alzheimer's Disease Is Diagnosed — or Even Suspected

Alzheimer's Disease is more widespread than you *think*. You probably already know a handful of people with Alzheimer's—although you may not even realize they have it. In fact, many people who have Alzheimer's may not be aware they have it.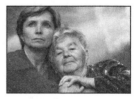

One of those Alzheimer's sufferers may be a member of your family— or perhaps a close friend.

> **FACT:** One out of five people over age 65—and 50% of people over age 85 are afflicted with Alzheimer's Disease. At least **5.2 million Americans and 26.6 million people** worldwide currently suffer from the disease. In 2010, there

were **454,000 new cases** in America alone, and nearly one million new cases annually are expected by the year 2050.[9]

Why should you care about this?

Because Alzheimer's disease is a family illness. Those who are afflicted with the disease do not suffer alone—every member of the family suffers as well. In fact, Alzheimer's is the one disease that can single-handedly **bankrupt** all but the wealthiest families, and devastate the entire family— not just financially, but also physically, psychologically and emotionally.

Until there's a cure for Alzheimer's, there are effective strategies you can use that can enable you to successfully manage the disease and rise above its adverse effects on your family.

Here are four crucial steps you can take to protect yourself from the emotional, physical and financial devastation caused by Alzheimer's Disease.

➢ **Step 1: Create a plan.** Even before Alzheimer's Disease is diagnosed—or even suspected—you must have a plan of action in place that will keep you moving forward so that you don't sink into despair or helplessness. When you have a step-by-step roadmap, you'll be better able to handle the diverse aspects of being a caregiver to someone with Alzheimer's.

For example, you should put in place immediately **two legal documents**—containing three essential items that will help **eliminate the risk of losing your life savings, your retirement plan and all your assets, including your home** in the process of caring for your loved one.

➢ **Step 2: Prepare in advance to avoid the devastating mistakes that Alzheimer's caregivers commonly make.** These mistakes include the failure to make the necessary preparations on a timely basis, and, as a result, NOT qualify for financial assistance from the government. Other common mistakes include:

• The incorrect titling of assets

---

[9]U.S. Food and Drug Administration Website; *2012 Alzheimer's Disease Facts and Figures*, http://www.alz.org/downloads/facts_figures_2012.pdf

- Not knowing how to communicate properly with your loved one, which can lead to unnecessary emotional outbursts and unmanageable behavior

- Not knowing when and if you should seek home care or admit your loved one into a nursing home, and

- Not knowing how to pay for it without going broke.

Any one of these—and many more common mistakes—could cause irreparable harm to your own health, your finances, and your life.

➤ **Step 3: Educate yourself about Alzheimer's Disease**—the key aspects of care-giving, and all the options that are open to you. If you are like most Alzheimer's caregivers, you've probably done your share of jumping from one website to another looking for information about Alzheimer's that is scattered all over the Internet. This is the WRONG WAY to educate yourself.

Why? Because much of the information you'll find online might seem to make sense to you, or even appear useful—but in actuality, there is a lot of erroneous and inaccurate information, half-truths and factoids on the Web masquerading as the truth. If you base your actions upon such information, it will cost you dearly in the long run. Don't be a do-it-yourselfer when it comes to being informed about caring for an Alzheimer's care-giving sufferer. Rely only on authoritative information.

There's a **little-known network** of care-giving advocates, health-care experts, financial planners, legal advisors and everyday people who've successfully managed all the care-giving aspects of Alzheimer's. They have spelled out in simple terms all the right strategies that will make you feel confident that you're doing the right thing for your loved one and yourself every step of the way.

There is a **secret** to safeguarding your emotional, physical and psychological health—and even your sanity—as your loved one's Alzheimer's Disease progresses. This little-known secret is used by many successful Alzheimer's caregivers to help them rise above the harsh reality of Alzheimer's in the family and finding the strength, the sense of humor and the hidden blessing behind it.

➤ **Step 2: Take action.** If you learn only one thing, let it be this: Not taking meaningful action is the worst thing you can do. Because once

Alzheimer's disease is officially diagnosed, it's already at an advanced stage, and it may be progressing rapidly.

The key to successfully coping with Alzheimer's in your family is to accept the things about Alzheimer's Disease that you cannot change, and to manage the parts of Alzheimer's care-giving that you CAN control. http://undergroundhealthreporter.com/vitamin-e-

Permanent Blindness: An Epidemic!

Few people realize that macular degeneration is the leading cause of blindness in men and women aged 55 and over. It affects more than ten million people in the United States alone—and millions more all over the world.

Age-Related Macular Degeneration (AMD) is a condition which causes light-sensitive cells in the back of the eye to stop functioning, resulting in *severe vision loss*. AMD affects the *middle part of the visual field*, which is needed for driving as well as many other everyday activities.

In January 1997, Dr. Carl Kupfer, then the Director of the National Eye Institute, National Institutes of Health, stated publicly that macular degeneration will soon take on aspects of an epidemic!

This is alarming news because according to a recent poll, **Americans dread blindness more than any other disability**.[10]

The picture below on the left shows what a grid looks like with normal vision. The picture on the right shows what the same grid might look like in the eyes of someone suffering from AMD.

---

[10]American Macular Degeneration Foundation
Macular Degeneration Foundation,
http://www.charity.com/printer_macular_degeneration-charityofthemonth.shtml

Unfortunately, there is currently no cure for AMD. However, there is a way to drastically slow down the progression of this incurable disease. The National Eye Institute says there is only one proven way to slow down the progression of AMD once diagnosed. That one way is through **vitamin supplementation**.

AMD is a real problem with real consequences when left untreated. A recent study done at the University of Wisconsin showed that exercise may reduce the risk of developing AMD. The study tracked 3,874 men and women (aged 43 to 86) over a fifteen-year period. The study concluded that those with an active lifestyle were **70% less likely to develop the degenerative eye disease** than those with a sedentary lifestyle. For this reason, it is recommended that:

- If you are not currently exercising, you talk to your physician about starting a healthy exercise program.

- If you, like many of us, do not exercise regularly—or have not exercised three to five times per week over the last fifteen years, then it's even more important that you take a macular degeneration supplement.

The antioxidants that are found in an amazing supplement called Preserve Mac Forte have been **proven by the National Eye Institute to slow the progression of AMD and possibly help prevent blindness**.

Although most people don't believe they will ever go blind, AMD actually affects many middle-aged people these days, and it is predicted that an ever-increasing number of individuals will develop it every year as more and more "baby boomers" approach age 55 and beyond.

Dr. Warren Ringold has successfully treated hundreds of patients suffering from AMD, and has recently developed the only proven and established method for treating AMD, slowing its progression and reducing the serious risk of permanent blindness.

A New Form of CoQ10 Can Make You Younger

Dr. Tatsumasa Mae, a renowned doctor of biomedicine, who's widely acknowledged as the *world's leading CoQ10 researcher*, recently conducted a study comparing the **anti-aging properties** of the conventional form of CoQ10 with a new, highly absorbable form called Accel CoQ10.

The results of this study were **nothing short of miraculous!** Dr. Mae studied three groups of laboratory mice:

Group 1: Mice taking no CoQ10.

Group 2: Mice taking conventional CoQ10.

Group 3: Mice taking the new "super-absorbable" Accel CoQ10.

After a few months, all the test mice from Group 1 died of natural causes—and they all exhibited typical signs of oxidative stress.

The test mice from Group 2, who were taking conventional CoQ10, were still alive, but they showed some signs of aging. These mice lived longer than those that took no CoQ10, but they died from similar conditions.

The test mice from Group 3, who were taking Accel CoQ10, showed the most **astonishing** results. They were not just alive—they actually *looked younger* than the mice in Group 2!

The Accel mice also had more energy. They ran around in their cages with all the vigor of mice half their age, and they were able to run continuously on their treadmills for *two and a half times longer* than mice from Group 2. In spite of being "old" (for mice), they showed almost **no signs of aging**. After a year, the "super mice" on Accel **aged 22% more slowly** than mice taking conventional CoQ10.

This may quite possibly be **the most critical health discovery since Dr. Karl Folkers first identified CoQ10 back in 1958**.

If you're like most people, you probably don't mind getting older "in years." What you do mind is the progressive deterioration of your body, the loss of youthful energy, and looking older as you age.

But what if you could:

- ✓ Feel as **energetic as a teenager** well into your 60s and 70s?

- ✓ Slow down the aging process, **reduce wrinkles** and protect your skin from the photo-aging effects of sunlight?

- ✓ **Strengthen your heart** and have better cardiovascular health?

- ✓ **Improve your memory** and enhance your ability to learn?

- ✓ Have **clearer vision**, healthier gums and bronchial health?

- ✓ Enable your body to **burn fat** more effectively?

- ✓ Retain the power of youth well into your old age?

If you could do all of these things, I'm betting you wouldn't mind getting older, would you?

And that's exactly what is possible with Accel CoQ10. This new form of CoQ10 is **eight times more potent** than the conventional store-bought CoQ10 and has already been shown to **slow the aging process by up to 51%!**

CoQ10 has rightfully been one of the most celebrated nutrients of the past few decades. Some people even claim it's a *medical miracle*. But sadly, hordes of people who have flocked to health food stores to buy CoQ10 became disillusioned when they started taking the supplement and found out **it doesn't work!**

That's because most brands of CoQ10 sold on the market are the oxidized version; that is, they use an inexpensive form of the enzyme called ubiquinone. When you take ordinary CoQ10 pills, before it can begin working, your body has to reduce the compound to ubiquinol—**the most biologically active form of coenzyme Q10**. Only then can it absorb the CoQ10 as a nutrient that can power your cellular metabolism.

As you grow older, your body progressively loses the ability to reduce Ubiquinone, and when you're over the age of 50, your body is no longer able to absorb this form of CoQ10 at all. When this happens, CoQ10 never makes it to your cells—consequently, you get none of the benefits!

Accel CoQ10 has been reduced to ubiquinol before you ingest it. This eliminates the need for your body to reduce it, and enables you to absorb Accel directly into your bloodstream where it can do you the most good.

This is not just a theory or hopeful speculation. The science behind this new discovery is *published* and *peer reviewed*. The health benefits of Accel are **scientifically validated**.

So, although there's nothing you can do to stop the hands of time, there is something you can do to stop the havoc that time wreaks on your body. Instead of becoming increasingly slow, weak and feeble every day—you'll crank up your body's ability to produce energy. You'll also be able to keep the mental and physical abilities you've enjoyed all your life—and even look younger—simply by taking one caplet of this new form of CoQ10 a day.

For more details about Accel, go to the following webpage: http://www.alsearsmd.com/2010/01/the-awful-truth-about-coq10/

Arthritis

World Famous Doctor Reveals Non-Drug Cure for Arthritis

Dr. Stephen Sinatra, M.D., stunned the medical establishment and the world recently when he announced a **non-drug cure for arthritis** and the **world's first non-surgical joint replacement for arthritis**.

This makes one wonder which is more stunning—the news that a natural cure has been found for the prevalent (and previously incurable) disease of arthritis or the news that a world famous medical doctor actually prescribes this natural cure instead of the usual drugs for arthritis pain and surgery for joint replacement!

In any event, arthritis sufferers all over the world are breathing a collective sigh of relief—*pain relief*, that is—over this breakthrough discovery that could put an end to their arthritis woes forever.

Even arthritic individuals whose cartilage has been damaged (or is completely gone) have reason to rejoice. It used to be said that **once damaged, cartilage can never heal**. When knee cartilage is damaged, for instance, it's a progressive degenerative condition. The person loses more cartilage every day until it is completely gone; the knee hurts 24 hours a day; and the only effective treatment—until recently—was knee replacement surgery.

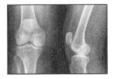

Now, with Dr. Sinatra's startling discovery, **knee and joint replacement may well become obsolete** and completely unnecessary. His natural cure has been shown to repair and even **rebuild cartilage**!

You can see before-and-after x-rays and CT scans that PROVE that arthritis is healing and repairing itself by going to Dr. Sinatra's website: http://undergroundhealthreporter.com/r/arthritisinterrupted/

This is an **ingeniously easy plan**. I recommend it to anyone with arthritis who is concerned about the dangers and side effects associated with drugs and painkillers.

–Brendan Montano, MD

...this has become my "go-to" reference book for state-of-the-art information on the holistic and nutritional treatment of arthritis. Even if you don't have arthritis, you should read this book! **Absolutely brilliant!**

—Johnny Bowden, PhD, CNS, author,
The Most Effective Natural Cures on Earth and
The Most Effective Ways to Live Longer

Dr. Sinatra is one of the very few board-certified doctors with advanced degrees in nutritional science. Prior to his discovery, the only remedies for easing the pain of arthritis and improving the flexibility and mobility of arthritis sufferers were:

> **Glucosamine supplements:** But most glucosamine supplements DON'T contain the *correct form* of glucosamine (the one used in the majority of clinical tests) nor the proper dose used in those trials.

> **Fish oil capsules:** Most arthritis sufferers take a dose designed to halt ARTERY inflammation. Joint inflammation is much tougher and requires a much LARGER dose! (You must make sure you are taking enough.)

> **NSAID drug pain-relievers:** Yes, these do reduce the pain—but in the process they also BLOCK your body's ability to manufacture new cartilage. Result? Your cartilage-repairing supplements actually become counterproductive to arthritis relief.

> **Your diet:** Although you try to "eat right," studies show that even the most health-savvy individuals unknowingly consume foods and beverages that trigger **painful inflammation** in their joints and vertebrae.

> **Arthritis Healing super foods:** Most people with arthritis and degenerative back problems AREN'T eating enough of these super foods to really nourish and repair damaged cartilage and disks.

Arthritis has always been a very *stubborn*—and *incurable*—condition —until now.

Merely taking a little fish oil or glucosamine may give you modest relief, but this isn't enough to REVERSE the destruction of your joints and spine—or trigger their HEALING.

To truly conquer this stubborn condition you need a "shotgun strategy" that blasts arthritis at every level—the **molecular, biochemical, nutritional, physical** and **emotional/psychological** levels. And that's exactly what Dr. Sinatra's remarkable new arthritis cure does! I'm delighted to recommend this to you. In fact, it would be a disservice NOT to tell you about it because this solution can relieve so much needless suffering.

The results are truly impressive. Most orthopedic surgeons will tell you it is NOT possible to heal arthritis. That's because medical schools teach doctors that painkilling drugs and joint replacement are the only "treatments" for arthritis.

But here's what one surprised orthopedic surgeon reported after examining one of the people who tested Dr. Sinatra's new "shotgun strategy": "This patient displays a **remarkable recovery**. His x-rays show new cartilage where there was none just one year ago."

This is the closest thing to a true cure for joint and back problems we have today. And I want you—and all your friends who are suffering right now—to know about it because **"once you stop moving, you start dying."**

That old adage is absolutely true. Inactivity due to arthritis triggers a domino effect that leads to overweight, cardiovascular problems, incomplete circulation, toxin accumulation, metabolic disorders, and **accelerated aging**.

Doctors generally don't consider arthritis to be life-threatening, but it definitely shortens your life and keeps you from enjoying every moment of your life.

Don't let arthritis shorten your life or the life of a loved one by even a single day, Or to rob you of the joy and pleasure this wonderful life offers when you stay active and pain-free.

For additional articles on natural remedies to heal Arthritis go to:
http://undergroundhealthreporter.com/health-conditions/arthritis

Why Joint Pain Pills Don't Work —
And What Does

Drugstores sell an assortment of pills that are supposed to relieve aching joints. Many of those pills contain the popular nutrients *glucosamine* and *chondroitin*.

Glucosamine and chondroitin have been popular for years among those who suffer from the **debilitating joint pain, swelling** and **inflammation** of osteoarthritis, rheumatoid arthritis and gout. What most people don't know, however, is that although glucosamine and chondroitin do provide some of the building blocks your body needs to create new joint cartilage, they have absolutely no effect on the real cause of your joint destruction.

Did you know that **the erosion of cartilage (which leads to joint pain) is caused by your own immune system?** Yes, it's hard to believe but it's your own body that's destroying your cartilage.

In fact, even though glucosamine and chondroitin may knock out your joint pain temporarily, they actually *contribute to the breakdown of cartilage!*

Here's how that happens: Your immune system works hard to protect you against toxins that find their way into your body and build up in your joints. When it senses the presence of the toxic enzymes that are slowly eating away at your joints, your immune system goes into overdrive. It is actually this heightened immune system response that creates the **stiffness** and **inflammation** in your joints that cause you pain. Your heightened immune response starts working against not just the toxic enzymes but your healthy joint tissue as well.

Before long, scientists came to realize that glucosamine and chondroitin could never rebuild cartilage unless something stopped the immune system from scavenging your own joints. After more than a decade of research, they isolated a molecule that works with your immune system— keeping it in perfect balance and putting a stop to the destruction of your joints.

Ten clinical trials on humans have been conducted on this molecule at a cost of over **$45 million**. The molecule can only be harnessed through a *proprietary extraction process* that is protected by fourteen U.S. patents! This makes it the most exclusive, clinically validated and effective natural supplement for joint pain ever made—one which literally *halts the breakdown of cartilage* and throws it in *reverse*.

Cancer

Billion-Dollar Drug Company Hides Astounding Discovery of a Natural Cancer Cure

10,000 Times Stronger than Chemo — but without the side effects!

One pharmaceutical company actually made the *"discovery of the century"*—a **miracle breakthrough** that could save you or someone you love from the ravages of cancer.

But they **hid the secret for seven full years**—with no plan to tell anyone about it ever!

What if you found out that a company discovered a *cure for cancer*—and kept that information *hidden* from the public for seven years? I would consider that an **outrage!** After all, according to the United Nations, cancer had become the **leading cause of death in 2010**. And millions of people all over the world have died from it when their lives could have been saved. According to the United Nations Cancer Research Agency, cancer **will kill more than 13.2 million people a year by 2030**. That's almost double the number who died from the disease in 2008.

How many people do you know who died from cancer in the past seven years? I'm sure you're asking yourself, "Why would a company suppress information about a cure for cancer and deliberately allow millions of people to die?" The reason they hid the discovery was that the substance they found is completely *natural* so they couldn't take out a patent on it and, therefore, they couldn't make any money from it!

Go to http://undergroundhealthreporter.com/gravioladigest to read the full story of this astounding breakthrough—and the dozens of other underground cures not yet available to mainstream medicine.

Diabetes

Doctor-Recommended Drug-Free Diabetes Remedy with a 100% Success Rate

> **I have never had one single patient that I have not been able to get off of their diabetes medicines.**
>
> –Dr. Stefan Ripich

Dr. Stefan Ripich may become the doctor most hated by the mainstream medical establishment—if he isn't already. That's because he's discovered the most inexpensive, natural, drug-free remedy for one of the 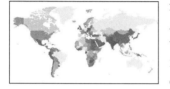 most prevalent diseases of our time—diabetes. Approximately **27% of the American population** (81 million people) and more than **170 million people worldwide** suffer from diabetes or pre-diabetes.

And unlike other doctors who avoid disseminating news about natural cures (for fear of ridicule from colleagues in the medical industry), Dr. Ripich is sharing his discovery with anyone who cares to listen.

Because he is an outspoken proliferation of this natural approach to diabetes, Dr. Ripich could single-handedly threaten the multi-billion dollar diabetes cash cow. Since he has 100% success rate in getting his patients completely OFF diabetes meds and related drugs, what would happen to the diabetes industry if diabetes medications were to become totally obsolete?

That, of course, would be good news for the tens of millions of people worldwide who suffer from diabetes, but bad news for the members of the pharmaceutical and medical industries whose livelihoods depend on people's dependence on diabetes medications.

Do you see why Dr. Ripich is bound to become very unpopular among his fellow doctors very soon?

Contrary to popular belief, **diabetes can be reversed!**

This mantra is echoed by Dr. Christian K. Roberts, the lead researcher of a clinical study on diabetes conducted at the UCLA School of Medicine. The UCLA study found that Type 2 patients were able to completely **reverse their diabetes in just three weeks** by using a simple, inexpensive, utterly safe, non-drug approach, which corroborates Dr. Ripich's contention.

More recently, a multicenter clinical research study of the Diabetes Prevention Program (DPP) showed this same approach to be **twice as effective** when tested head-to-head against Glucophage, today's leading glucose-lowering drug for Type 2 diabetes.

"Diabetes is curable and reversible," says Dr. Ripich. "You can manage your life and your diabetes without medications. Your body has enormous power to heal itself if you get yourself in a position for that natural healing power to flow. It's easier than you think."

Dr. Ripich has recently made available to the public a day-by-day, step-by-step guide that has been proven to reverse Type 2 diabetes and pre-diabetes in 30 days or less—and it even shows people with Type 1 how to dramatically reduce their insulin dose.

Some Type 1 diabetics who had blood sugar levels between 400 and 450, and who were using 40 to 65 units of insulin per day have been able to dramatically lower their insulin by 80% to 12 units a day!

A five-minute eye-opening video shows how Dr. Ripich has been able to virtually eliminate his patients' risk of deadly diabetic complications, such as heart attack (which is responsible for 75% of all diabetes-related deaths).

You can view it at: http://undergroundhealthreporter.com/r/0-30cure/ and get the full story about Dr. Ripich's 30-day diabetes cure.

The Life-Changing Discovery
that's Turning Conventional Blood Sugar
Advice Upside Down

Three years ago, a monumental study changed the way the world thinks about managing blood sugar.

That study's objective was to find out how a specific medicinal mushroom affects glucose metabolism. For centuries, the mushroom (called *Agaricus blazei*) had been used for just about *everything else*—from stress relief to strengthening the immune system and supporting healthy cholesterol levels. But the study conducted three years ago was the very first time a study demonstrated the mushroom's powerful ability to support healthy blood sugar levels.

So stunning were the results of the study that they shattered conventional wisdom about controlling blood sugar. It was shown unequivocally that maintaining healthy blood sugar is not just about what you eat—or DON'T eat—or how much you exercise.

Researchers found that when subjects took 1500 mg of the mushroom extract daily, it actually ***boosted the body's adiponectin levels***. Researchers theorize that having higher adiponectin levels means your body can stop working overtime because it can clear sugar from your blood quickly and efficiently—just the way it's supposed to.

This means you may be able to:

- No longer limit yourself to a "sugar free" diet

- **Eat what you want, when you want** (without going overboard, of course)

- Stop feeling guilty when you're unable to follow your doctor's long list of "dos" and "don'ts"

- Finally get rid of those nasty mood swings

- Turn your body into a lean, mean, carb- and fat-burning machine —and consequently shed excess weight, and

- Have *plenty of energy* to get through the day—without feeling like you're running on fumes.

This medicinal mushroom is one of the ONLY things that has been shown to have the ability to help keep your body's adiponectin level where it needs to be.

As extraordinary as the results of the study have been, the mushroom's blood sugar support ability has been largely unknown to most people because it's a secret that no one is talking about.

Dr. Allan Spreen, who for many years had been working with patients who were concerned about their blood sugar, found himself *frustrated* and disheartened when the medications and "diet and exercise" advice he was giving to his patients didn't work. Therefore, he was ecstatic when he recently discovered the promising effects of the medicinal mushroom.

But he also learned that when *Agaricus blazei* was combined with the *lightning-fast* blood support properties of a cucumber-shaped gourd (which families in India have been eating for generations), the results were even more impressive. One of the early animal studies involving this gourd found that it outperformed other traditional blood sugar supporting herbs dramatically—and produced **effects that started within one week**.

A brand-new, double-blind, placebo-controlled human trial by the makers of the standardized gourd extract found in this supplement showed downright *remarkable results*. By the end of the trial, the gourd group's blood sugar had improved by leaps and bounds, **dropping by as much as 18%**—while the placebo group had a *7% increase*.

WARNING: Lowering Blood Sugar to Curb Diabetes Can Increase Risk of Death

What mainstream medicine has been telling us for years about diabetes is completely **wrong!**

You've heard it said before—and most doctors routinely recommend it —keeping your blood sugar (or blood glucose) under control is one of the most important measures you can take to avoid diabetes.

And if you already have diabetes, reducing your blood sugar can delay the onset of complications.

Even the American Diabetes Association tells us that this is the best Way to treat diabetes. Yet, a recent study published in *The New England Journal of Medicine* shows unequivocally that lowering blood sugar is not good medical advice. In fact, it's **downright dangerous!**

The study proves conclusively that lowering your blood sugar as a way of managing diabetes can **increase your risk of death**. The ACCORD study consisted of 10,000 diabetic patients. The initial plan was to study the effects of intensive therapy to lower their blood sugar. The patients were monitored, and their risks of heart attack, stroke, and death were assessed.

The researchers were *surprised* by the results. Patients who had lowered their blood sugar levels the most were at higher risk of death. In fact, the study came to an abrupt halt because it was found that as blood sugar levels dropped, more patients had heart attacks—or **died**.

Why has the medical establishment fallen for the *myth* that lowering blood sugar is the key to managing diabetes? Here's why: it's because, once again, they are focused on the *symptoms* and not the cause of the disease. High blood sugar is just a *symptom* of diabetes. The true cause is **spiked insulin levels**, which is a result of insulin resistance.

Unfortunately, typical treatments make the problem worse. That's because they're designed to increase insulin levels in the body, in order to deal with the elevated blood sugar.

As the ACCORD study proves, this is a mistake. The best way to treat diabetes is to **improve your body's sensitivity to insulin**. The ideal way to do that is through your diet. Here are four simple tips you can follow:

1. **Eliminate heavily processed foods.** This means any kind of junk food, including fried and sugary foods. They help fuel diabetes and keep it alive. Practically all of these foods are high-glycemic, which means they spike your blood sugar and, as a result, your insulin levels. Also, if it's packaged and comes in a box or bag, chances are it's not good for you. Packaged food always come with multiple ingredients, including hydrogenated oils (trans fats) to give it a long shelf life.

2. **Eat more protein.** Your focus should be on eating foods that have one or two ingredients. That means getting the bulk of your calories from protein. Good sources are grass-fed beef, free-range chicken, organ meats, and wild-caught fish.

3. **Eat healthy fats.** Make sure to get healthy fats in your diet, too. Great sources are wild-caught salmon, olive oil, almonds, avocados, and egg yolks.

4. **Get plenty of fruits and veggies.** The majority—if not all your carbs—should come from fruits and vegetables. Eat fruits with the skin intact, as it provides a good source of fiber. Stay clear of

starches, grains, and any other kind of carb that's been heavily processed.

Most diabetics think they're stuck with the disease for life. That simply isn't true. Type-2 diabetes can be reversed. And it all starts by changing your diet, starting with these four simple tips.

But there's more to it than that. You can read the full story in *The Diabetes Reversal Report*. This guide tells you the secret ingredients for triggering the healing ability that's in every cell in your body. You'll get an easy-to-follow plan that puts you on the right path for treating diabetes. You can get a copy of *The Diabetes Reversal Report* by going to: http://undergroundhealthreporter.com/Diabetes-WARNING

Heart Disease

Surefire Strategies for Lowering Your Blood Pressure and Protecting Yourself from a Heart Attack or Stroke

One in three adults over the age of 20 have high blood pressure. All too often, the very first symptom of heart disease is an actual heart attack.

Heart disease sneaks up on you like a thief in the night. And far too many adults—most of whom never even suspected that they had *high blood pressure*, high cholesterol or clogged arteries—become victims of a heart attack or stroke.

"Every 37 seconds, an American dies of heart disease." According to the American Heart Association, about **65 million Americans over the age of 20 have high blood pressure**. That's about one in three adults. In 2003 more than 52,000 Americans died from complications related to high blood pressure. Between 1993 and 2004 the rate of death from high blood pressure rose nearly 30 percent.

Heart disease—not cancer, Alzheimer's, diabetes, the flu or pneumonia —is the No. 1 cause of death, killing an average of 2,400 Americans every single day. Yet, that need not happen to you because there are specific strategies that can **reduce your risk of getting a heart attack to zero.**

Interestingly, these strategies have little to do with following the doctor's orders or popping a few pills; in fact, often, those courses of action still lead to serious coronary events. Sadly, by the time most people find this out, it is too late.

Do You Have High Blood Pressure?

Only 63% of those with high blood pressure are even aware they have it, according to the American Heart Association.

If you don't know what your blood pressure is, you can have it checked at your doctor's office or at a health clinic. Or if you want to avoid a high-stress visit to a doctor's office or health facility, there are drugstores such as Walgreens and Rite-Aid that have BP monitoring devices on premises that you can use for free.

Better still, for as little as $15, you can buy a blood pressure kit that enables you to check your own BP at home any time you want. Once you get a BP reading, check the table below to see where you stand.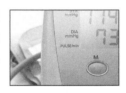

Blood Pressure Stage	Systolic	Diastolic
Normal	<120	<80
Pre-Hypertension	120-139	80-99
Stage One Hypertension	140-159	90-99
Stage Two Hypertension	160+	100+

Whether you are in pre-hypertension, Stage 1 or Stage 2 hypertension, there are natural treatment options and alternative remedies that you can use to reduce your blood pressure. Your doctor will probably never tell you about these options because he or she may be unaware of their existence.

The Wonders of Lecithin

Lecithin is a phospholipid that is part of cell membranes. It consists primarily of the B vitamin choline, as well as linoleic acid and inositol. Commercial lecithin can be extracted from egg yolks or soybeans. The type derived from soybeans (called *soya lecithin*) is generally used as an emulsifier in the manufacture of chocolate. It increases the chocolate's flow properties (fluidity) by reducing viscosity. Without lecithin, chocolate is dense and thick and tends to have a rough surface because it keeps the air bubbles inside the bar.

Similarly, lecithin acts as an emulsifier in the human body, helping it disperse fats and protecting the vital organs and arteries from fatty buildup. It also helps improve liver function and repair cell membranes; aids in the absorption of thiamin by the liver and Vitamin A by the intestine; and promotes energy.

Scientific studies have shown that lecithin has the ability to break up cholesterol into small particles— and, thus, prevent it from building up against the walls of the arteries and veins.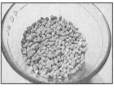

Using lecithin granules or capsules as a dietary supplement is just one of the many strategies you can employ to control high blood pressure.

Dead of a Heart Attack ... at the Age of 47!

Craig Anderson learned the horrors of uncontrolled high blood pressure *the hard way*. While he was still in college, his father who was only 47 years old died of a heart attack.

Fast forward years later: Craig was married and had kids of his own when he found out that he had **Stage 2 hypertension**, with a BP of 170/100. He was *shocked, horrified* and filled with the *overwhelming fear* that he was quickly going down the same deadly path that had killed his father many years earlier.

More than anything, he dreaded the thought of dying of a heart attack or stroke and leaving his wife without a husband and his kids without a dad. He vowed to take better care of his health and investigate all the ways he could avoid the deadly fate of his dad.

As he looked into it, he faced an even **bigger shock**. He discovered that **conventional medical treatments for high blood pressure were even worse than the disease**! The only options offered by mainstream medicine were things like diuretics, beta blockers, alpha-blockers and vasodilators— all of which came with side effects and health risks that were undesirable and, in some cases, life-threatening.

The worst part was that drugs taken to reduce blood pressure were, at best, a *temporary fix* because they treated only the *symptoms* of high BP and not the cause—and came with an **exorbitant price tag**!

Craig set out to find a cheaper, more effective, more permanent and more natural way to lower his blood pressure. After months of research, he finally discovered the perfect strategy. When he implemented it **his BP reading plummeted almost 50 points down to 113/80**!

And the best part was that by using nothing but natural remedies and treatments, his blood pressure dropped dramatically. No drugs. No side effects. And no exorbitant cost.

To find out the simple steps Craig took not just to significantly reduce his blood pressure, but also to keep his blood pressure firmly under control for the rest of his life, go to: http://undergroundhealthreporter.com/bloodpressurekit

Craig's foolproof solution is something anyone—even you—can do to normalize your blood pressure, regain heart health and finally have the peace of mind that comes from knowing that you can virtually protect yourself from having a heart attack or stroke.

Chapter 11 - The Healing Power of Your Mind

How Thoughts Prevent and Heal Disease — Including Cancer!

What is a thought? A thought is a form conceived in the mind. It consists of a few micro-miliwatts of energy flowing through the brain. It is estimated that **the average human being has 60,000 thoughts a day**.

Since thoughts come and go rapidly, and are as transitory as passing clouds, most people dismiss them as *unimportant* and *inconsequential*. Nothing could be further from the truth.

Thoughts wield a powerful impact on your body, your health—and your life. "Every good thought you think is contributing its share to the ultimate result of your life," Canadian author, Grenville Kleiser, once said. Likewise, every negative thought you think contributes its share and is capable of wreaking havoc on your health, whether you realize it or not. **A Single Thought Has the Potential to Produce Over a Million Dollars' Worth of a Cancer-fighting Chemical!** To understand how this works, consider the following story:

One afternoon in late spring, Dan and Robert visited a theme park with their families. Both were in line to ride the park's most thrilling roller coaster.

Dan and Robert are very much alike. They are the same age, have the same upbringing, grew up in the same town; they even went to the same high school back in the 80s.

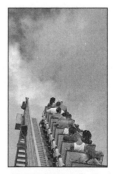

But there is a *difference*. Dan loves thrill rides, and while he's on the roller coaster, his thoughts are saying, *"This is fun!"* Robert, on the other hand, is secretly terrified of thrill rides, and when he's on the roller coaster, his thoughts scream, *"This is terrifying!"*

The roller coaster ride is over in a few minutes, but both Dan and Robert are unaware that their health has been affected more than they can imagine.

141

Robert's only thought while on the ride was of *terror*. That thought caused his body to produce massive quantities of **cortisol, adrenaline** and other substances that **shut down the immune system**. It might not be immediately apparent, but that one roller coaster ride caused a chemical imbalance that is likely to make Robert physically, emotionally or psychologically ill later in life.

Dan's only thought, on the other hand, while riding the roller coaster was that of *exhilaration*. That thought caused his body to produce **endorphins**, which contain the powerful **cancer-fighting chemicals** *interleukin* and *interferon*. If you were to buy the anti-cancer drug Interleukin-2 (manufactured by Chiron Corporation under the brand name Proleukin), a full course of treatment would cost you **upwards of $40,000**—and it would be accompanied by a long list of the side effects.

Which would you rather do? "You could take that joy ride," says Deepak Chopra, M.D., and **make a million dollars' worth of Interleukin-2**." Or live in fear and potentially damage your immune system?

The Phenomenon of Spontaneous Healing

Perhaps you've heard of people suffering from incurable, often lingering, disease or sickness who were healed spontaneously and restored to perfect health—without any medical intervention whatsoever.

This phenomenon of spontaneous healing, which some people liken to a *spiritual or religious experience*, is often explained by the body's miraculous ability to manufacture chemicals that heal the body.

For example, when you think thoughts of tranquility at a deep level of awareness, your body—specifically, your leukocytes, adrenal cells and macrophages—start producing a **tranquilizing biochemical** similar to diazepam (a drug usually referred to by its trademark name, Valium). Unlike the Valium manufactured by Hoffman-La Roche, the tranquilizing chemical produced by the body is the "real diazepam"—the molecule of tranquility, which supports the proper functioning of the immune system.

A negative thought, on the other hand, releases a cascade of harmful chemicals, which take their toll on your health and well-being, slowly kill your spirit, and may also lead to physical disease.

How You Can Counteract Negative Conditioned Responses

Consciously directing your mind to think only thoughts that cause the body to produce health-enhancing biochemicals is, quite frankly, easier said than done. That's because we are made up of **conditioned** reflexes, which automatically react to people and circumstances producing very **predictable biochemical outcomes**—behavioral outcomes—and ultimately, physical outcomes.

Therefore, if you, like Dan, are *conditioned* to enjoy roller coasters, your positive thoughts would cause your body to produce substances that are **beneficial** to your health. If, on the other hand, you, like Robert, are conditioned to fear roller coasters, your negative thoughts would cause your body to produce substances that are **detrimental** to your health, and may even cause illness.

No two people process the same stimulus in the same way. That which causes fear in Robert obviously does not affect Dan in the same way. The difference in the way you or another person reacts to stressors—and the difference in your ability (or inability) to relax and experience tranquility —has to do with your conditioning.

To counteract conditioned responses that may be detrimental to your health, you can choose to *reframe* those stressors in ways that neutralize their negative effect. By far, the most effective method for overcoming deep-seated conditioning is **hypnosis**.

Through hypnosis, which is a focused state of attention that increases suggestibility, you can rise above conditioned reflexes, adapt easily to stressful situations, resolve anxieties, and create positive ways of looking at the world. These go a long way toward releasing the body's innate ability to produce health-enhancing biochemicals superior to any that a pharmaceutical company could ever manufacture.

How to Use Your Hidden Healing Power
to Erase Disease, Pain and Sickness
at *Amazing* Speeds

You may not realize it yet, but you were born with an *awesome* ability to heal. It's a healing power that resides in *every human being*—but most people will never know they have it. You are about to learn how to put this astonishing hidden talent to use.

It involves a healing method that enables *you* to literally heal disease, illness, pain, trauma, emotional distress, and suffering—without drugs or medication or devices. All by yourself!

This is not some *mystical* healing method that produces hit-or-miss results—but something so **potent** that doctors from the famed Mayo Clinic are actually studying it! In fact, Neil Kay, M.D., a doctor at the Mayo Clinic, calls it "a much simpler and yet easily applied **alternative medicine for cancer patients**."

Other medical doctors have called the results they've seen this healing method produce **"absolutely remarkable"** and **"phenomenal."** Dr. Bill Manahan of the University of Minnesota Medical School calls it **"equal in importance to the incredible discoveries in the forties called *anti-biotics* and in the fifties called *immunizations*."** Even health expert and bestselling author, Deepak Chopra, M.D. holds this healing phenomenon in high regard.

So what exactly is it?

It's a method that involves simple body movements, controlled breathing and focused attention. It was developed by a remarkable healer and teacher, Master Chunyi Lin, whose healing techniques have been studied by over *45,000 people* all over the world.

Master Lin insists that everyone has the same healing ability that he has—and that same ability is just waiting to be unleashed in you.

How James Conquered Brain Cancer

Four and a half years ago, James suffered a grand mal seizure. Doctors discovered a tumor the size of a tangerine in James's brain—malignant and **cancerous**.

Surgeons removed 75% of the tumor, and chemotherapy and radiation burned the cancer into remission. Last year it returned with a vengeance. Doctors gave him **three months to live**, maybe six months with chemotherapy.

He chose chemotherapy, which incapacitated him within a month. Soon thereafter, he found the healing technique taught by Master Lin, and within hours of practicing it, the pain was gone. "I was literally skipping down the hall and down the stairs. I couldn't believe it," James said.

That was a year ago. Today, James feels better than he has felt in five years. The tumor has shrunk, and the doctors are *astounded* that James is still alive.

You, too, can heal yourself and fill yourself with boundless energy—and you can help your friends and relatives heal themselves. You don't need to be a doctor to help others heal.

If you or someone you know suffers from cancer, AIDS, diabetes, heart disease, arthritis, hypertension, depression, anxiety, emotional distress, respiratory disease, allergies, migraines, problems with reproductive organs, back pain, blood disorders, liver disease, fibromyalgia, or even **weight issues**, you must read the free booklet about the effective healing technique that can help alleviate any health problem.

Terminal Bone Cancer, Type 2 Diabetes, a Lump in the Breast — Vanish Instantly!

Among the stunning stories you'll find in the free booklet are the personal accounts of Dr. Ron Jahner (naturopathic doctor and board certified acupuncturist with offices in Chicago and Santa Barbara, California). His father had terminal bone cancer and was told he had only a few weeks to live. That's when Dr. Jahner and his family became interested in learning Master Lin's healing technique. Today, because of Master Lin's teachings, his dad is alive and well—years after he was told he was going to die.

Seeing this result, Dr. Jahner then began treating many of his patients using the same healing technique. One of his patients was a seven-year-old girl who suffered from uncontrolled Type 2 diabetes. After Dr. Jahner performed one session of Master Lin's healing technique on her, and her blood sugar **tested perfectly normal**—something that had never happened before!

You can also read the story of Stacy Langager, a 22-year-old woman who suffered from fibrocystic breast disease. She had a **lump in her breast the size of a golf ball**. She sought the help of Master Lin. After the first treatment, **the lump was reduced by 95%**—down to the size of a pea. After the second treatment, the lump was *completely gone*.

To discover the amazing healing effects of this practice go to: <u>http://undergroundhealthreporter.com/qigong</u>

New Science Reveals How Pre-Programming Dreams Can Cure Your Mind and Body — *While You Sleep!*

Have you ever been somewhere and felt like you had been there before; or have you ever meant to call an old friend and, before you do, the friend calls? Has there ever been a time when an answer to a problem you've been trying to solve suddenly appears out of nowhere, or a nagging pain just "goes away"?

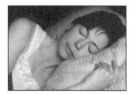

New research on the unconscious mind has revealed that these types of coincidences and sudden appearances do not happen by chance. Rather, they are often the physical manifestations of what our mind "works on" while we dream.

Researchers found that what you dream and what takes place in your physical world are indeed interrelated. It's more than just *déjà vu*, it's the **dream state affecting the physical state** and vice versa.

Taking this discovery one step further, researchers tested the theory that one could "pre-program a dream" in order to influence the mind to manifest something one needed or desired in the physical world.

The results of the research were astonishing because they found that:

> **The impact of a specific dream has physical, chemical, electromagnetic, psychological and psychic repercussions to that individual.** If you program your dreams for specific structures or events, they will materialize given that you focus on a single-minded desire ... such as curing the body or

solving a problem. These "healing dreams" are brought on by repetitive self-suggestion prior to sleep.

The study proved conclusively that dreams can be one of the greatest natural therapies. There is a growing body of science that asserts that dreams can be manipulated to control your body and environment in as little as one night.

By learning how to pre-program your dreams, you can create your personal, physical and health environment—and your Inner Self can cure your own mind and body.

> The inner senses have an electromagnetic reality and the mental enzymes act as sparks, setting off inner reactions. In the dream state these reactions are easily triggered. A destructive attitude can be changed overnight in the dream state because the whole electromagnetic balance has been changed ... **A powerful dream has the potential to completely eradicate a serious illness overnight**.
>
> –Jim Francis, Chief Research Advisor, Mind Surge

In the same way, dreams can completely reverse moods of depression, the urge to smoke, the inability to lose weight, or any harmful health condition—just by pre-programming up the necessary dreams. Dreams of this nature can be consciously evoked at will—in a surprisingly simple manner.

The researchers have provided practical examples in an informational report on pre-programming dreams. Here are some of them.

If your problem has something to do with:

- A need to improve your general feeling of wellness, you would repeat over and over, **"I will have dreams tonight that make me feel fit, well and bursting with energy."**

- Your desire to lose weight, then you would repeat over and over, **"I will have dreams tonight that cause me to become aware of my calorie intake and lose weight naturally."**

- If your problem is that you want to feel less stressed during the day, then you would repeat over and over, "**I will have dreams tonight that cause my stress level to reduce drastically so I feel calm and peaceful all day.**"

The report goes on to say that you can also "program up dreams where you are wealthy, happy and surrounded by friends. This will eventually 'break through' into your physical life and start to improve your personal situation," including the financial, social, or relationship aspects of your life.

It has been shown that **health improvement is one of the easiest and most effective types of dreams to pre-program**. The technique requires a little more than just repeating words before retiring, but it has resulted in almost miraculous health improvements in as little as twelve hours.

You can learn the complete dream programming technique in a free e-book titled *Mind Surge: The Consciousness Revolution*. In this one-of-a-kind e-book, you'll discover how to **cure your mind and body while you sleep as well as how to heal people across the world with the power of your mind**. (The book comes with a Remote Influencing exercise you can use immediately.)

You'll also learn how to attract luck, attract the ideal partner, and even beat casinos at their own game—all with your mind!

Go to http://undergroundhealthreporter.com/mindsurge to get the free e-book now.

Melt Away Disease Using Nothing More than Your Fingertips

There's a new frontier in healing that doesn't involve the use of pharmaceutical drugs or conventional medical treatments. It's called energy medicine, and it is a branch of alternative medicine that focuses on the use of the human energy field for healing.

Energy medicine is gradually becoming mainstream. Even Dr. Mehmet Oz, known as "America's Doctor" declared on The Oprah Winfrey Show and in his #1 *New York Times* bestseller, *You*, that energy medicine is a legitimate and effective healing modality, and the next big frontier in medicine.

The Healing Codes, discovered by Dr. Alex Loyd in 2001, employs energy medicine at its quintessential best. It involves using the fingertips of both hands to point toward one or more of the four different energy centers of the body, which nobody knew existed until Dr. Loyd discovered them.

The science behind *The Healing Codes* is compelling. When you employ the healing codes on yourself, the *internal stress* caused by **cellular memories** (which are believed to be the cause of 98% of all disease) completely disappears. And when that internal stress disappears, so does the disease. This has been **scientifically proven** through the use of Heart Rate Variability, the only reliable medical apparatus for measuring stress in the nervous system.

Here's a little background: Cellular memories, as the name suggests, are memories that have imprinted themselves in the cells. They are the result of life experiences. Stored in the cells of any human being, they almost always are the result of traumatic experiences from early childhood (or beyond). These cellular memories are like little transistor radios transmitting destructive energy patterns throughout the body, causing disease, chronic pain and, most important, **shutting down the body's immune system**.

"Our best hope for healing incurable illness and disease in the future might very well lie in finding a way to **heal destructive cellular memories**," states Dr. John Sarno, professor at the medical school at New York University, who goes on to say, "If you can heal that cellular memory, then the illness or disease or chronic pain is very likely to heal."

That's exactly what *The Healing Codes* do. When you use your finger-tips to point at one or more of the four energy centers in the body (there's a specific code for every disease), you effectively clear the destructive cellular memories from your body and, in doing so, you turn your immune system back on. "And when your immune system is working correctly, it's impossible to get sick," says Dr. Alex Loyd.

Even if you're already sick, once you remove the internal stress caused by those destructive cellular memories, your immune system will begin to function the way it's supposed to—and **there's nothing the body is not capable of healing**.

Ever since *The Healing Codes* were discovered, **miraculous cures** have become an everyday occurrence among its thousands of users all over the world. Every known disease has responded well to this natural therapy—including so-called incurable diseases like cancer, AIDS and Lou Gehrig's Disease. The Healing Codes organization has amassed hundreds of pages of testimonials from people who have cured themselves of diseases ranging from acid reflux, diabetes, heart disease, arthritis, herpes, emphysema (and even uterine fibroids) to psychological problems like anxiety or clinical depression.

> Mark Victor Hansen, the celebrated best-selling author of the *Chicken Soup for the Soul* series of books, whose cousin was healed miraculously of cancer after using *The Healing Codes*, was prompted to say,
>
> > Dr. Alex Loyd has the defining healing technology in the world today—it will revolutionize health. It is the easiest way to get well and stay well fast. Dr. Alex Loyd may very well be the Albert Schweitzer of our time!

The beauty of *The Healing Codes* is that anyone—even a child as young as seven—can self-administer the simple healing technique at home in as little as eight minutes.

The "Invisible Commercial" — How The Media Uses Subliminal Advertising to Hypnotize You

Perhaps you're not aware of it, but every single day, you're being hypnotized without your consent.

What's worse is that you're being manipulated to do *things*, believe ideas, and make decisions that other people want you to do, believe and decide.

As a society, our lives are centered on media—such as television, cinema and advertising—that we unwittingly allow to permeate our subconscious. The shows we watch on television, for example, shape the way we think—more than we are willing to admit. TV influences the way we process information, the way we make decisions, what we believe we can or cannot achieve, and our concept of what is possible and not possible.

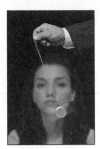

Breaking Through a Performance Barrier to a New Level of Human Possibility

For many centuries, scientists and athletes alike believed it was impossible to run one mile in less than four minutes. But on May 6, 1954, Roger Bannister crossed the finish line of Oxford's Iffley Road track, completing the mile in 3 minutes, 59.4 seconds— becoming the world's first athlete to achieve such a feat.

In an interview, Bannister stated, "There was a mystique, **a belief that it couldn't be done**, but I think it was more of a *psychological barrier* than a physical barrier."

Curiously, just six weeks later, John Landy broke Bannister's record with a 3 minute 58 second finish. Since then, the four-minute barrier has been broken by many male athletes. The current record is held by Hicham El Guerrouj, who ran one mile in 3 minutes and 43.13 seconds in Rome in 1999.

People are truly capable of **transcending ordinary human limitations**, but only if they believe it is *possible*. Mass media contributes to the global population's *limited* view of what is possible and impossible.

"Television is a mass hypnotist to the global mind," declares David Icke, public speaker and author of sixteen books. He cites experiments, which show that electrical signals in the subconscious mind respond to stimuli 1½ seconds before the conscious mind even begins to take action. TV installs beliefs in our subconscious mind every minute. Once those beliefs are installed (without our *conscious cooperation or permission*), our lives begin to be governed by those beliefs—whether those beliefs are right or wrong.

Dr. Bruce Lipton, bestselling author of *Biology of Belief* and former cell biologist at Stanford Medical School, states that **wrong beliefs cause 90% to 95%of all illness and disease**. Wrong beliefs include things like,

✓ "I'm never going to amount to anything"

✓ "Something bad will happen"

✓ "I am unlovable"

✓ "People are out to get me."

They are our *unconscious programming.*

Television, cinema and *advertising* contribute significantly to that programming. Often, **subliminal messages** are deliberately embedded in TV shows, movies and advertisements that we, the viewing public, consume. Thus, we unconsciously allow ourselves to be exposed to messages that quite often *disempower* us or even *wreak havoc on our health*. Note: Subliminal messages are **suggestive messages that reside below the threshold of conscious perception**.

The First "Invisible Commercial"

In 1957, a market researcher named James M. Vicary began testing subliminal advertising in a New Jersey theater. The tests ran for six weeks, during which time, 45,000 movie-goers attended the theater and became unsuspecting subjects of the experiment.

The test consisted of inserting subliminal frames containing the words, "HUNGRY? EAT POPCORN" and "DRINK COKE®," within the reels of a feature film titled *Picnic* starring William Holden and Kim Novak. While the movie was playing, the subliminal messages went by so fast (1/3000th of a second) that the members of the audience didn't consciously see the words.

According to Mr. Vicary, the moviegoers' subconscious minds perceived the suggestions and, as a result, the "invisible commercial" caused Coke® sales to increase by 18.1% and popcorn sales surged by 57.7%.

Program Your Own Mind

What if you could use such powerful subliminal technology to "advertise to your own mind" have your desires manifest at an unprecedented speed? What if you could use subliminal messages to not only **defuse the**

negative programming (such as scarcity, inadequacy, hypochondria, victim syndrome, poverty consciousness, poor self-image, etc.) that was instilled in your subconscious mind by years of unfiltered exposure to TV, movies and the media but also **install empowering affirmations** into your subconscious?

Affirmations are undeniably a powerful tool for manifesting desires, especially when fueled by repetition. But they work only if your conscious mind does *not* contradict your affirmations. Here are a few examples of how your conscious mind blocks the power of your affirmations:

Your affirmation says...	Your conscious mind might be saying...
I am in perfect health.	Cancer runs in my family. I'll probably get cancer, too.
I earn a high 6-figure income.	I'll never earn that much. I'm just not smart enough.
I am in the best shape of my life.	I hate my body. Who am I kidding?
I am now attracting a loving soul mate to me.	I always attract the wrong kinds of people.

This is just one instance where the Emotional Freedom Technique, also called *meridian tapping*, is tremendously helpful. Tapping combines the dual modalities of ancient Chinese acupressure and modern psychology.

When you tap on the meridians (the circuitry within the body through which your life energy flows), an electrical signal is emitted that clears the *blocks in the subconscious mind*. This alters how the conscious mind responds to your affirmations, thereby making it all but certain that your affirmations will manifest into reality.

Transform Your Life
Take a Music Bath...

> Take a music bath once or twice a week
> for a few seasons. You will find it is to
> the soul what a water bath is to the body.
>
> —Oliver Wendell Holmes

Masaru Emoto, a creative and visionary Japanese researcher, observed that water reacts positively or negatively to different external stimuli—including *music*. This led him and his colleagues to conduct experiments to see how such stimuli affect the molecular structure of water.

In specific experiments, he placed glass bottles containing untreated, distilled water between two speakers and then played various kinds of music—for several hours. Next, he froze the water and photographed the molecules using a special microscope camera. He found that the type of music the water was exposed to influenced the molecular structure of the ice.

The ice formed from water that had been exposed to *classical music* resulted in beautiful, **snowflake-like** crystalline structures while the water exposed to music containing frenetic vibrations, such as *heavy metal music*, resulted in **distorted** and randomly formed crystalline structures.

Since the average adult human body is composed of over 70% water comprises, Emoto surmised that **music has the ability to alter the structure of molecules in the body**, thereby healing and transforming the body.

The curative power of music has given birth to a global community of registered music therapists, who utilize music to soothe, stimulate and support the development or recovery of abilities lost to illness or injury. A research study conducted at the Cognitive Brain Research Unit of the University of Helsinki in Finland found that the recovery rate of stroke victims who listened to music for one hour a day or more was significantly faster than those who didn't listen to music. *Memories and fluency of speech improved more rapidly*; music listeners appeared to have a more *cheerful* disposition and *focused attention*; their ability to control and perform mental operations and resolve conflicts **improved by 17%**—and their verbal **memory improved by 60%**.

Neuroscientists are convinced that music can help rewire a brain affected by illness or injury, but they're still trying to uncover the scientific basis for music's healing power. What they do know is that **music literally moves within us**.

Music travels through the brain's auditory cortex directly to the limbic system, the part of the brain responsible for emotional responses, hormonal secretions, motivation, pleasure, and pain.

Researchers are finding that music can be an effective remedy for those who suffer from various ailments.

- Music has been shown to **unlock memories** (at least temporarily) in Alzheimer's patients who have lost their recollection of most details of their lives.

- Music with rhythmic quality has been shown to help Parkinson's Disease sufferers by **activating the brain's motor regions to restore the ability to walk**.

- Music's predictable beats have also been shown to initiate speech in those with speech impediments (such as stutterers)—and make their *halting speech patterns disappear.*

Other afflictions that have responded to music therapy include autism, reading disabilities like dyslexia, and even impaired growth in premature babies.

You might wonder, if music has the ability to alter a molecule's structure, unlock memories, cause disabilities to disappear, restore motor skills and improve brain functions, could it also reduce *stress* and *pain*, banish illness, generate feelings of *well-being*, **create the relationships you desire**, accelerate your ability to achieve *success* and *abundance*, and *enhance your spiritual growth?*

The answer to those questions is "yes!"

Renowned composer Paul Hoffman and Paul Scheele of Learning Strategies have created music called *Sonic Access*, which **immediately transforms the state of your brain**. Electroencephalograph (EEG) studies show that the brain waves of people who listen to the **specially created**

audio template of *Sonic Access* instantly change! Beta spikes drastically diminish and alpha waves significantly increase. Brain wave patterns rich in alpha waves create the preferred state for personal development and long-lasting change.

It is now possible to harness music's amazing power to positively affect your physical, emotional, and mental well-being—and transform every area of your life.

Simply by listening to the Sonic Access CDs containing this *technologically advance*d music, you can:

- Affect your thinking, perception, and memory—as well as every organ in your body;
- Activate your energy field, or chakra center, levels;
- Automatically slow your breathing and heart rates and bring your brain waves into an ideal state;
- Clarify your intentions to achieve your greatest success and wellbeing;
- Access your higher intelligence;
- Tap into your body's complex energy field, which can give you powers beyond what others have to achieve goals;
- Create new neural connections between your right and left brain hemispheres to significantly improve your learning capabilities; and
- Help heal your body.

To learn more about music's amazing power to transform your life go to http://undergroundhealthreporter.com/take-a-music-bath

How to Unlock Your Inner Genius

What if you could get "into the head" of any expert or genius in any field of endeavor and actually view your situation, opportunity, or problem from the expert's point of view—and get **genius answers** to any of life's perplexing questions?

That would be like having people like Albert Einstein, Sir Isaac Newton, Leonardo da Vinci, Thomas Edison and Galileo Galilei (to name a few) doing your thinking and making your decisions for you!

Many neuroscientists say that **human genius resides in a dormant part of the brain** and, therefore, is rarely used. Others say the **vast untapped human potential** lies in the *unconscious mind.*

Most of us have experienced moments of brilliance; maybe you've had moments like these:

- You wrote an essay, poetry or letter that was so **riveting** that you hardly recognized the writing as yours;

- **You solved a personal or business problem** with startling creativity and the greatest of ease—at a time when no one else could find a solution...

- You came up with a seemingly random idea that made you, your family or your company **more money,** or made you **more productive** with minimum effort;

- You delivered a speech without any written notes—and **dazzled everyone in the audience**—even though you normally have stage fright and aren't good at making speeches;

- You gave a performance **worthy of a standing ovation** in a play, recital or debate—but you couldn't duplicate that stellar performance when you tried to do it again;

- You **uttered the right words at exactly the right time**—and those words changed people's lives, maybe even your own.

If any of these things have happened to you, you may have dismissed it as *pure luck*, or a *momentary flash of inspiration*. You probably had no idea where it came from. Or you might have just dismissed the entire event as a *fluke*—never again to be repeated.

Actually, those events are *glimpses* into your own hidden genius. What *amazing and mysterious powers* might be hiding in the underutilized part of your brain and your unconscious mind?

There is a way you can experience those *moments of brilliance* at will. You can actually tune into those secret messages that your brain automatically sends you, and, as a result, **boost your IQ, solve any problem, accelerate learning, recognize golden opportunities, and supercharge your intuition.**

That way is called "Image Streaming." It is revealed in a remarkable CD course called *Genius Code* created by mind development pioneer Win Wenger, Ph.D. and Paul Scheele.

Image Streaming is a simple, elegant mental technique that anyone can learn quickly and easily—and **get a "genius" answer to any question in as little as one minute!**

There is even an Image Streaming process called "Borrowed Genius," which allows you to get into the head of any expert or genius in any field and get genius answers to your dilemmas, opportunities or situations.

Your brain is like an ultra-intelligent professor babbling at the speed of light. It streams out images, thoughts, and impressions—seemingly random, completely unceasing, often distracting—yet those random images (sometimes referred to as "stream of consciousness"):

- Contain brilliant insights and innovative solutions
- Lead to rapid learning and super brain waves—things that you would normally not have access to in your everyday level of awareness.

Chapter 12 - Add Nourishment
with Super Supplements

Three Superfoods that
Deliver Super Nutrition

If you're like most people, you've been told to "Eat your fruits and vegetables" since you were a child. Mainstream media including the *New York Times, Los Angeles Times*, health and fitness publications, National Public Radio, as well as countless university studies have long proclaimed that a diet rich in vegetables and fruits can increase your energy levels ... boost your immune system ... reduce your risk of illness ... and recharge your body.

However, although fruits and vegetables are indeed good for your health ... eating them is no longer good enough to promote optimum health and wellness. Here's why:

Vegetables and Fruits That Are Conventionally Grown
Are Nutritionally Depleted – and
May Even be Hazardous to Your Health

1. Today's produce is significantly lower in essential nutrients than foods produced 50 years ago because modern farming practices have depleted our soils of minerals. Depleted soils yield nutrient-poor produce. You now need approximately 10 servings of vegetables and fruits to obtain the nutritional equivalent of 1 serving from 50 years ago.

2. The long shipping and storage time between harvest and market degrades the nutrient content further. As a result, most vegetables and fruits sold in commercial establishments are nutritionally depleted.

3. The use of pesticides and other chemical additives in non-organic farming yield nutritionally deficient produce that may have long-term health risks.

4. An estimated 80% of food crops (ranging from corn, tomatoes, alfalfa to sugar beets) are now genetically engineered. These genetically modified (GMO) crops have had their genetic material altered using genetic engineering techniques. Genetically engineered produce have been shown to cause serious health problems in those who consume them.

The first-ever long-term study of the health effects of GMO foods (conducted at the University of Caen in France) shows that a lifelong diet of genetically modified foods causes tumors, organ damage and premature death in lab mice.

Multivitamin Supplements Are <u>Not</u> the Solution for Promoting Long-Term Health and Wellness

According to the world's largest study on multivitamins, people who take multivitamin supplements are not gaining health benefits. Instead, most of the vitamins and minerals are excreted, thereby earning them the nickname of "expensive urine."

That's because this is the way vitamin and mineral supplements are made: The nutrients in foods are isolated and extracted, and put into a synthetic chemical structure that the body does not recognize as food. Synthetic vitamins often have an entirely different chemical structure from those found in food.

> "Taking multivitamins doesn't solve the problem —it is impossible to capture all of the vitamins, minerals, disease-fighting [nutrients] ... in a pill."
>
> – *Source: National Cancer Institute*

While there are several types of food-based multivitamins and minerals on the market, many health authorities consider three super foods the ideal supplements, especially for those who are not able to consume a sufficient amount of organic fruits and vegetables each day.

Super Food No. 1: Spirulina

Spirulina is a blue green algae, which is considered **the most nutrient dense food on the planet**. It contains concentrations of nutrients far exceeding any other known vegetation. It is the best source of vegetable protein, containing about 65 % protein—higher than any other natural food —far more than animal flesh (20%), eggs (12%), whole milk (3%), soybeans (35%), peanuts (25%), or grains (8 to 14%). It is considered a *complete protein* because it contains all the essential amino acids.

Spirulina grows so fast that it yields twenty times more protein per acre than soybeans. It also contains extraordinary concentrations of vitamins, minerals and other nutrients, such as beta carotene (ten times more concentrated than that of carrots), iron, potassium, magnesium, copper, calcium, chromium, manganese, phosphorus, selenium, zinc, essential trace minerals, and gamma-linolenic acid. It is also the most abundant source of Vitamin B-12, and is also **rich in phytonutrients** and functional nutrients that have a demonstrably positive effect on health.

Because spirulina's nutrient profile is more potent than that of any other food, plant, grain or herb, it is considered a superior whole food alternative to isolated vitamin supplements. In addition to its contribution to the body's nutritional needs, it has been shown to be effective in the treatment of **cancer, high cholesterol, allergies, anemia, elevated blood sugar, cardiovascular diseases, viral infections, inflammatory conditions, liver damage** and **immunodeficiency diseases**.

Super Food No. 2: Chlorella

Chlorella is a single-celled, water-grown algae that contains more health-enhancing chlorophyll per gram than any other plant. It is extremely rich in vitamins, minerals, amino acids, essential fatty acids and many other nutrients that are beneficial to your health.

Chlorella also has an abundance of nucleic acids, which have powerful rejuvenating properties that slow down the aging process, keeps the skin looking youthful and wrinkle-free, and helps you have a longer life.

Dr. Benjamin S. Frank, author of *The No-Aging Diet and Nucleic Acid Therapy in Aging and Degenerative Disease*, treated his patients with foods rich in nucleic acids, and reported that such a diet made his patients look and feel 6 to 12 years younger than their chronological age, and their over-all health dramatically improved. They also experienced a substantial fading of lines and wrinkles, and developed healthier, younger-looking skin after only 2 months.

Super Food No. 3: Moringa

The moringa is a genus of trees indigenous to Southern India and Northern Africa, and now cultivated in Central and South America, Sri Lanka, Malaysia and the Philippines. The leaves of the species called *moringa oleifera*, have become recognized in recent years as being highly beneficial to human health.

Moringa leaves are an anti-aging powerhouse because they contain **several thousand times more of the powerful anti-aging nutrient zeatin** than any other known plant. A study published in *Rejuvenation Research* shows the undeniable *youth-preserving* effects of zeatin because of its ability to induce cell division and growth, and *delay cell aging*. With the zeatin contained in moringa, new skin cells grow at a faster rate than old skin cells die. This results in a **marked reduction of wrinkles** on the face and other parts of the body, and a **more youthful skin appearance**.

Moringa leaves also has 90 essential nutrients and 2 compounds that **prevent cancer and reducing tumors** (or retarding their growth). This has earned moringa the reputation of being a cancer preventative plant. India's natural Ayurvedic medicine uses moringa leaves to prevent and treat over 300 diseases.

A Bureau of Plant Industry report states that, gram per gram, moringa leaves contain: twice the protein content of 8 ounces of milk (and 4 times the calcium); the Vitamin C equivalent of 7 oranges; the potassium content of 3 bananas; 3 times the iron of spinach; and 4 times the Vitamin A of carrots.

How to "Drink" Your Superfoods Everyday

If you're among the 70% of adults who aren't getting their recommended daily servings of vegetables—and the thought of eating ten servings of spinach, collards, kale, green beans, peppers, and other green vegetables doesn't sound appealing (or possible for you to do)—you have the option of taking spirulina, chlorella and moringa instead.

Quantum Wellness Botanical Institute of Beverly Hills has formulated **the ideal blend of not only these three powerful superfoods, but five more of the most nutrient-dense superfoods on earth**. All you have to do is mix a scoop of this powder blend in a glass water, juice, or your favorite smoothie—and drink it every day. In the time it takes you to pour yourself a cup of coffee, you can supply your body with mega-nutrition, energize and revitalize your entire body, support your immune system, and achieve optimum health and wellness.

To discover the "Mega-8 Superfoods," which include the **world's greatest anti-aging superfood** ... the best superfood for **rejuvenation and cancer prevention** ... a superfood that contains **600 times more Vitamin C than oranges** ... a super herb with **spectacular health benefits more prized than gold** ... and **"the most antioxidant-rich superfood on the planet,"** go to: http://www.MegaNutritionOrganicsuperfood.com

Take a Vitamin Pill and Never Get Sunburn or Skin Cancer

If you enjoy being out in the sunshine but worry about getting a **sunburn** and increasing your **risk of skin cancer**, there are groundbreaking studies that show that taking a *specific vitamin pill* can protect you from the damaging effects of sun exposure—without the use of sunscreen.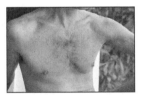

This nutrient enables you and your family to spend whole days in the sun without giving a thought to sunburn or skin damage—and it doesn't block the sun's beneficial rays, so your body can benefit from the Vitamin D produced by sun exposure.

Your Sunscreen Could Be Causing Skin Cancer!

In the past, if an average person wanted to be out in the sun for more than just a few minutes, he or she would have to slather greasy (and often smelly) sunscreen all over their body. But given the recent news that **four out of five sunscreens could actually be hazardous to your health**, you have probably been rethinking the use of sunscreens.

According to reports released by the Food & Drug Administration (FDA), **more than 80% of the more than 800 sunscreens tested** in recent years contained potentially dangerous chemicals and cancer-causing agents. Some of the biggest culprits contained in commercial sunscreens are Benzophenone, homosalate, octyl methoxycinnamate (also called octinoxate), octyl-dimethyl-PABA, and 4-methyl-benzylidene camphor. These hormone mimickers can compromise the entire immune system, leaving your body susceptible to a number of diseases, including cancer.

But that's not all. Some sunscreens contain Padimate-0 and parsol 1789 (also known as avobenzone), which have been linked to DNA damage. This, of course, can have a detrimental effect on your skin cells and their ability to rejuvenate and repair themselves, which can result in *premature aging*.

Dioxybenzone and oxybezone, two common ingredients in the most popular sunscreen brands are some of the most powerful free radical generators known to man. This means that these ingredients, when absorbed by the skin can actually intensify free radical damage, causing cells to break down and illness to ensue. This breakdown is believed to either **allow melanoma cancer cells to generate in the deep layers of the skin** or to actually cause them. Either way, a link between these dangerous chemicals and deadly skin cancer has been established.

What makes the problem even worse is that when sunscreen is slathered onto the skin, it is very easily absorbed into the bloodstream, causing damage to various parts of the body—*not just the skin*. This year alone, more than 3.5 million new cases of skin cancer will be reported across the United States. From mild carcinomas to deadly melanomas, skin cancer is a real danger to all of us.

Because most sunscreen products contain toxic chemicals that could cause you more harm than good, how can you protect yourself from sunburn, skin damage and cancer?

Studies Show an Antioxidant Pill Gives 800% More Sun Protection than Sunscreen

Al Sears, MD, has discovered a way to **change the way your skin responds to sunlight** and halt the harmful process that leads to burns, wrinkles and aging—at the cellular level.

Three clinical studies show conclusively that when a "sunscreen pill" (containing a very powerful antioxidant) was taken by individuals with varying degrees of hypersensitivity to the sun, they experienced a **higher tolerance to sun exposure** and a significantly **lower tendency to redden, flush, or have sun-induced skin irritation**.

Everyone who participated in the three studies started to see results within two or three days. Even among those with the palest (i.e., most sun sensitive) skin, there was *800% more sun protection*. It was like having an "internal sunscreen." And the best part about this "**internal sunscreen**" is that it works without blocking the sun's rays. According to a recent study published in *Anticancer Research*, getting a little sunlight every day—about twenty minutes for fair skinned people, and two to four times as much for dark-skinned people—can r**educe the risk of sixteen types of cancer** in both men and women.

There's no question that your body has a physical need for sunlight, which causes your skin to produce Vitamin D, which has been clinically proven to:

✓ Halt or even reverse the effects of bone diseases like rickets, osteomalacia and **osteoporosis**

✓ Prevent many types of cancers—including **prostate, breast** and **ovarian** cancer

✓ Reduce the risk of melanoma

✓ Elevate mood and *boost mental performance*

✓ Relieve depression and reduce the symptoms of schizophrenia

✓ Lower blood pressure

✓ Increase white blood cell activity and strengthen the immune system

✓ Reduce high blood sugar levels, increase insulin sensitivity and **prevent diabetes**

✓ Lower the amount of bad cholesterol in the blood

✓ Promote weight loss

✓ Provide more restful sleep

✓ Increase energy and vitality

To learn more about this vital vitamin and how to ensure adequate vitamin D levels, go to http://undergroundhealthreporter.com/5-minute-health-tip-take-a-vitamin-d-bath

When Doctors Feel Pain, This is What They Use

The idea of doctors feeling pain is a *paradox*. We seldom think of doctors as being in poor health—or in pain. Yet, doctors are as likely to experience pain as the average person—perhaps even more so because they are more often exposed to sick people than the average individual.

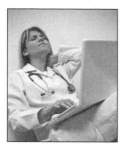

So what do doctors "in the know" do when they're in pain? Do they take the same pain medications that they routinely prescribe to their patients?

Some do. But the more savvy ones like Dr. Allan Spreen seek out effective solutions that have little or no side effects. Sometimes such pain remedies are not always available to the general public.

One of the "secret" pain relievers that has been available—but which only truly healthy-savvy people have been able to get their hands on—is *Soothanol X2*.

Soothanol X2 is the result of the work of a brilliant health expert named Jon Barron. For years, Barron had been researching a pain relief formula that could **erase virtually any kind of pain** on contact just by rubbing it on and would also eliminate the wait for pills to work.

Together with fellow researcher Ron Manwarren, Barron isolated eleven different cutting-edge botanical and organic compounds that all showed immense promise in relieving pain. Those compounds were emu oil, arnica oil, ginger, St. John's wort oil, MSM, lemonene oil, wintergreen, calendula oil, cayenne pepper, methanol and olive oil.

But they were missing an ingredient that would "deliver" all those compounds to the site of pain.

After extensive experimentation, they discovered a perfect substance that could dissolve the eleven botanical and organic compounds, move them rapidly to the site of the pain and penetrate to areas in the body that nothing else could reach as fast. That substance is DMSO. They named the product they created Soothanol X2.

Dr. H. Harry Szmant, Chairman of the University of Detroit's chemistry department, observed that DMSO **can speed up important chemical reactions "a billion fold."** As a result, you need only a drop or two of Soothanol X2 to feel incredible results.

Jon Barron and Ron Manwarren soon realized that their Soothanol X2 formula, which consisted of the eleven compounds and DMSO, was indeed the "holy grail" of pain relief for the following reasons:

1. It has the ability to **rub out pain on contact**.

2. Unlike commonly prescribed and over-the-counter pain pills, which take time to work, the application of one or two drops of *Soothanol X2* **delivers pain relief in as little as 45 seconds**.

3. There are **no known side effects**. Unlike the popular non-steroidal anti-inflammatory drugs (NSAIDs) such as Ibuprofen, naproxen sodium, ketoprofen and even aspirin—which all have adverse drug reactions ranging from cartilage breakdown, gastrointestinal and renal effects, and even congestive heart failure—Soothanol X2 has been shown to produce no side effects.

4. Its revolutionary "direct delivery" system neatly bypasses the entire digestive system, so it **won't upset the stomach** or **stress the kidneys or liver**.

5. There's never any need to worry about interactions with aspirin, blood-thinners or other pills you may already be taking.

One interesting phenomenon is that applying DMSO to one affected joint or area often leads to pain relief in some other part of the body. That's because DMSO has **systemic** effects, according to Dr. Morton Walker, author of *DMSO: Natural Healer*.

Clearly, DMSO is the cornerstone that makes the *Soothanol X2* formula a pain-relieving powerhouse unlike any other. It does what no pain pill on earth can do—and it does it safely and is non-addictive.

Chapter 13 - Sexual Chemistry

Pheromones: The Science of Sexual Chemistry

> Scientific studies have actually shown that subjects who used synthesized pheromones had sex more often.
>
> *–The Los Angeles Times*

> The power of smell is undeniable ... humans are influenced by airborne chemicals undetectable as odors, called pheromones. Researchers at the University of Chicago say they have the first proof that humans produce and react to pheromones.
>
> *–CNN*

> Pheromones can **improve one's sex life**, pheromones send out subconscious signals to the opposite sex that naturally **trigger romantic feelings**.
>
> *–McCall's Magazine*

ABC News recently reported that scientists at San Francisco State University found that women who added pheromone to their perfume reported a **more than 50% increase in sexual attention from men**. The study, which was published in the *Journal of Physiology and Behavior*, found that **74% of the women** saw an overall increase in three or more of 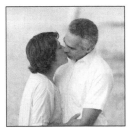 the following socio-sexual behaviors: frequency of dates, kissing, heavy petting and affection, sexual intercourse, and sleeping closer to their partner.

Sexual Magnetism magazine featured the findings of an Australian organization, **Bennett Research**, which conducted a survey of 306 men using pheromones. **Ninety percent (90%)** of them reported that their use of pheromones had increased their attractiveness to women.

They reported an increase in various socio-sexual behaviors, as follows:

- Making conversation — 61%;

- Starting up a conversation — 52%;

- Expressing an interest in the man — 43%;

- Being responsive to him — 40%;

- Paying unsolicited compliments — 36%; and

- Overt flirting — 34%.

Countless similar studies have since been conducted—and the results are consistently **mind-boggling**. Pheromones (particularly optimized pheromones) appear to have the ability to dramatically increase sexual attraction between men and women. This is why pheromones have sparked a stampede of eager buyers in recent years.

WARNING: The unprecedented interest in pheromones has also spawned an entire industry of unscrupulous pheromone vendors that **peddle worthless pheromone products**. *Let the buyer beware!*

Scientists have long been on the quest for the "perfect aphrodisiac." To date, the most perfect aphrodisiac ever discovered is pheromones. The reason will become obvious as you read on.

Why are pheromones called "secret seducers"—and how can they dramatically improve your love life?

Pheromones are chemicals that are secreted in our sweat (and other bodily fluids). Mammals and other animals also secrete pheromones, and scientists have long known that these pheromones are natural **sexual attractants** that wield a powerful influence on their **mating habits**.

> **It's not just the birds and the bees.** If you've ever observed the way a male animal is **irresistibly attracted** to a female in *heat*, you already understand the awesome power of pheromones in sexual encounters. Monkeys, grass carps, blue crabs and ants are just some of the animals that release pheromones as **enticements to love**.

Likewise, pheromones affect the mating habits of human beings. These **behavior-altering** chemicals are the driving force behind all sexual attraction. They **influence how often we have sex**—*and with whom*. Does this mean that when humans smell pheromones, we act like love crazed tomcats ready to pounce on any member of the opposite sex that happens to be nearby? Not exactly. The effects of pheromones on humans are more *subtle*, but, nonetheless, **powerful**.

Pheromones perform many tasks other than just **stimulating us to have sex**. They have been used as appetite suppressants, contraceptives and sedatives, and have also been used to regulate the menstrual cycles of women, as well as treat a host of illnesses, including impotence, sexual disorders and prostate cancer.

However, it is pheromones' **sexual attractant** properties that have captured the public's fascination—for obvious reasons.

Pheromones are **odorless**, and because they waft through the air in the smallest traces, they're barely perceptible. In fact, it is only through our vomeronasal organ (VNO) located in our nasal cavity that we're able to detect pheromones. Although pheromones cannot be seen, heard, smelled or touched, they *secretly* affect our biological processes, which, in turn, stimulate our sexual drives and reproductive behaviors. That's why they're often called "secret seducers."

When pheromones are optimized, they naturally release neurotransmitters that directly alter the behavior of the opposite sex—more particularly, they **trigger sexual excitement**.

Pheromones for Men vs. Pheromones for Women

Scientists have identified the chemical, androstenone, as the male pheromone. In addition to increasing the **animal magnetism** of a man, androstenones bring about an **increase in the luteinizing hormone (LH)** in a woman who happens to be nearby—thereby causing a woman to have a heightened sexual responsiveness to a man.

The compound, *copulin*, on the other hand, has been identified as the female pheromone. When optimized, copulins bring about a **testosterone surge** in men, thereby causing a man to have a heightened sexual responsiveness to a woman.

According to a recent report published in the London publication, *The Independent*, scientific research shows that by releasing female pheromones (copulins), women **may trick men into believing that that they are more attractive** than they actually are.

Among other things, users of optimized androstenones and copulins have reported that they had:

- Become seductive and desirable to the opposite sex

- More frequent sex

- Been able to attract the man/woman of their dreams

- Dramatically improved their sex appeal

- Been able to arouse romantic feelings in the opposite sex

- Been able to get more dates

- Gained a competitive edge in business affairs

WARNING: Not all commercially available androstenones and copulins are created equal. Pheromone vendors that carry optimized pheromones for men and optimized pheromones for women are rare. For optimized pheromones I recommend LuvEssentials (Lodix Corporation).

How to Bypass Your Conscious Mind and Program Your Unconscious Mind — While You Sleep

Question: What do Chaka Khan ... Dr. Louis B. Cady ... and Anthony Robbins have in common?

Answer: They all believe in the **awesome power of paraliminals** to make massive changes in their lives.

Paraliminals are a cutting edge self-improvement technology developed by Paul Scheele and Learning Strategies. Paraliminal recordings are applicable not just to psychiatric patients but also average people who desire optimum health, fitness and peak performance in life—without having to rely on will power or self-discipline.

Whenever you want to make a radical change to improve your life—and that change requires changing programmed opinions, self-defeating beliefs and behaviors that are hardwired within you—**it is a Herculean task**, to say the least!

That's because what you normally do is *make a **conscious** choice* to change yourself—either through will power or self-discipline.

No matter how you look at it, change is *difficult* to accomplish—whether you want to stop smoking, lose weight, improve your memory, gain new skills, overcome fear or anxiety, get rid of an addiction, improve your relationships, generate new behaviors or take your career to new heights.

But what if. . . instead of using will power or discipline, you could **bypass your conscious mind**, access your unconscious mind directly, and **reprogram it to create the long-lasting changes** in you ... *while you sleep?*

That's what paraliminal recordings do.

Unlike "subliminal" recordings that have *inaudible* programming messages embedded, "paraliminals" are recordings that actually enable you to distinctly hear the programming messages. The interesting thing about these professionally recorded audio programs is that they feature two programming messages being delivered to you in both ears, with two different trains of thought, simultaneously—and with gentle and relaxing music and white noise in the background.

The difference between this type of programming and "subliminals" is that, with subliminals, you never know if the programming message will enter your unconscious mind. That will depend on the threshold settings of the recording. With the paraliminal recordings, however, there is no doubt whatsoever that you are hearing the audio messages, because they are **audible**—and you can choose to listen to one channel or the other.

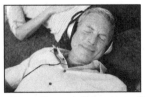

The magic of these audio programs is that if you relax and "drive your concentration right down the middle" of both of the simultaneous audio tracks, you can't pay attention to both at the same time and the messages—which are highly therapeutic—enter your unconscious mind, **bypassing the resistance of your conscious mind** altogether. Once you have control of your unconscious mind in such a manner, you're able to eliminate the conditioned, automatically trained behaviors and self-defeating emotional responses—and **easily install new behaviors in as little as 20 minutes**.

In the past, the only way you could even attempt to control your unconscious mind (which governs your opinions, beliefs, emotional states, and behaviors) is through in-depth psychotherapy, deep hypnosis, or relentless, repetitive self-reprogramming using multiple affirmations, multiply repeated, for a long period of time. And those things sometimes yield little or no results.

With paraliminal technology, all you have to do is:

- ✓ Select the aspect of your life you want to change;
- ✓ Pull out the paraliminal audio CD that corresponds to that desired change;
- ✓ Listen to the twenty-minute CD using headphones—and just *relax* or *sleep*, if you wish.

That's really all that's required to create the dramatic changes in your life that you couldn't accomplish before. That's also why doctors like **Louis B. Cady recommends the paraliminal CDs to his patients**, and an increasing number of health practitioners are doing the same. Even self-improvement leaders like Anthony Robbins and Jack Canfield highly recommend paraliminals.

Awakening Prologue:
A Mind-Boggling Experience

By Danica Collins[11]

About seven months ago, I came across a fascinating brain technology called Holosync® that people were raving about. I discovered that nearly *one million people in over 173 countries* had used it to make **startling** and **remarkable** improvements in their lives.

Bill Harris, who created this technology, had been researching mind-altering technologies for decades. He stumbled upon studies done by the Menninger Clinic, which determined the brain wave patterns of Indian yogis in deep meditation. He also came across a researcher at Mt. Sinai Medical Center in New York, who had discovered that those same brain wave patterns could be *induced* using **sound**, which meant that the deepest meditative states (and the incredible results they produce) could be experienced by anyone.

Thus began Bill's journey into the world of *binaural beat technology*. After years of experimentation, he developed a proprietary sound technology called Holosync®, which is available on a CD called *Awakening*

---

[11] Managing Editor, *The Underground Health Reporter*

Prologue, which contains binaural beats (embedded beneath soothing music and environmental sounds) that **slow down your brainwave patterns** into the alpha, theta, and delta ranges. Slowing down your brainwave patterns increases electrical fluctuations in your brain, changes the neural structure and pushes your brain to reorganize itself at higher, more complex levels of functioning.

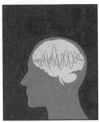

Once this happens, amazing mental, physical and emotional changes take place. Many researchers believe this is because different brainwave patterns are linked to the production of various neurochemicals associated with relaxation and stress release, *increased learning* and *creativity*, **memory**, and other desirable benefits.

The Holosync® website states that listening to the CD makes you **meditate as deeply as a Zen monk, literally at the touch of a button**. Meditating as deeply as a Zen monk delivers a multitude of benefits—not just for your health but for every aspect of your life. It's a proven fact that **people who meditate everyday are many times happier** than those who don't. They're also *healthier* and *live longer*. And, their sense of well-being is much higher than that of those who do not meditate.

> People who meditate are so much healthier that some insurance companies charge *lower premiums for people who meditate* than for the rest of the general population.

Meditators' minds are also sharper, and their *problem-solving abilities* are better. That's probably why many **high-powered executives, and even CEOs of Fortune 500 companies, make it a habit to meditate**.

When you meditate, your body manufactures an abundance of pleasure causing brain chemicals, such as endorphin and serotonin. When you meditate every day, your body creates these feel-good brain chemicals practically all the time.

People who meditate also have dramatically better mental health than those who don't meditate. They have *less anxiety*, anger, depression, and fear, and they have *better human relationships*, more friends, and feel much more *fulfilled* in their lives.

Anti-Aging and Longevity Linked to Meditation

Recent research performed by Dr. Vincent Giampapa, M.D., a prominent anti-aging researcher and past-president of the American Board of Anti-Aging Medicine, revealed that Holosync® dramatically affects production of three important hormones related to **increased longevity** and **enhanced well-being**; namely, cortisol, DHEA, and melatonin.

Cortisol is a hormone naturally produced by the adrenal glands. According to Dr. Giampapa, cortisol is the major age-accelerating hormone. It also interferes with learning and memory and is generally detrimental to your health and well-being.

Cortisol is the "stress hormone," and the more of it your body produces, the more stressed you feel, the more susceptible to disease you become and the faster you age! Meditation decreases cortisol levels, thereby reducing stress levels.

Another hormone, DHEA, is also produced by your adrenal glands. DHEA is a precursor, or source ingredient, to virtually every hormone your body needs. DHEA level is a key determinant of physiological age and resistance to disease. When levels are low, you are more susceptible to aging and disease; when they are high, the body is at its peak—vibrant, healthy, and able to combat disease effectively.

DHEA acts as a buffer against stress-related hormones (such as cortisol), which is why as you get older and make less DHEA you are more susceptible to stress and disease.

With All the Benefits of Meditation, Why Isn't Everyone Meditating?

Some people mistakenly believe that meditation is a religious or mystical ritual that goes against their faith. This is an incorrect assumption —meditation has nothing to do with religion or mysticism.

By far, the most common reason most people don't meditate because almost everyone who has tried to meditate has *failed miserably*. Often, people don't have the time, or their lives are so hectic that they are unable to put themselves in a state of stillness, or they get distracted by racing thoughts that ruin their concentration, or they tend to fall asleep during meditation.

For me, it was all of the above. That's why I was absolutely amazed when I loaded Holosync's *Awakening Prologue* CD into my CD player, put on my headphones, pushed the "play" button—and felt myself float into an incredibly deep meditative state almost instantly.

What was even more amazing was how I felt when I came out of meditation, which was completely at peace with the world. I had a new-found awareness and appreciation of people, places and things in my life; I experienced an incredible lightness of being; and I felt profoundly *happy*, as though everything in my life was perfect, and nothing could possibly go wrong. The best part is that feeling of being on top of the world lingered all day.

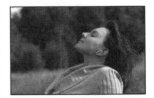

Imagine what you can accomplish in this world when you're feeling that way every single day of your life! And that's exactly what began happening in my life when I listened to the *Awakening Prologue* CD every day. My everyday stress was minimized; my **energy and productivity** reached levels never before attained; my **relationships improved** significantly; I was able to achieve goals more easily; I had a heightened sense of **well-being**; and I began achieving success in practically every area of my life. Furthermore, I noticed that I developed the ability to **solve problems more easily** and **learn new skills more quickly**.

I am convinced that people who listen to the *Awakening Prologue* CD everyday become empowered, renewed, rejuvenated and revitalized. They find their place in the world. They become more balanced, happier, healthier, more fulfilled—and their lives begin to function as never before.

To discover additional natural ways to practice mediation and reduce stress without spending a penny, go to:
http://undergroundhealthreporter.com/?s=meditation

Points on Your Outer Ear Can Help You Stop Smoking, Eliminate Pain and Heal Many Diseases

What if you could *touch* a single point on your ear and make your craving for food, nicotine, alcohol or any other substance **disappear**?

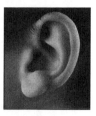

What if you could *massage* the helix point on the upper part of your ear and immediately **lower your blood pressure or reduce fever, inflammation or swelling**?

And what if you could *tug* on your ear lobe and **migraines** just vanished?

These scenarios seem like they come straight out of *fictional* films like *Bewitched*, in which characters tug at their ears or twitch their noses to cast magic spells. But the fact is healing the body through the outer ear is actually based on science, not fiction.

That science is auriculotherapy. Here's an excerpt from a book titled *The Amazing Science of Auriculotherapy*:

> Auriculotherapy (aw-RIK-ulo-therapy), also called auricular therapy, is a branch of alternative medicine that has its roots in traditional Chinese medicine. It is a state-of-the-art therapy for the treatment of over 350 diseases, and is a clinical science *recognized by the World Health Organization* and **approved by the Food and Drug Administration (FDA).**
>
> One of the core principles of this healing technology is that the outer portion of the ear (i.e., the auricle) is a *microsystem* that represents every part of the human body. In other words, every point of the outer ear corresponds to, and is associated with, a specific part of the human anatomy.
>
> Whereas general body acupuncture addresses health problems by working on the energy meridians of the body, auriculotherapy is based on **nerve connections** (in the human nervous system) and offers specific *localized treatment* for the organs or systems involved in the health problem.

Auriculotherapy has been used successfully for ...

- **Smoking cessation:** Auriculotherapy is thought to be seven times more powerful than other methods used for smoking cessation; a single auriculotherapy treatment has been shown to **reduce smoking from twenty or more cigarettes a day down to three to five a day**.

- **Allergies**

- **Weight Loss:** Clinical studies showed an average of **one to two pounds lost per week** just by applying acupressure on the Hunger Point of the outer ear.

- **Pain relief:** including back pain, headaches, neck pain, sciatica pain, radiating pain to arms or legs.

- **Sexual Stimulation:** Increases libido without dangerous drugs.

- **Hypertension**

- **Stress relief**

- **Insomnia:** A study involving 46 cases of insomnia—19 male and 27 female—was conducted in the *China Academy of Traditional Chinese Medicine* in Beijing. The test subjects were given auriculotherapy treatments. Of the 46 cases treated, 32 cases (69.5%) were cured—i.e., able to sleep more than seven hours; thirteen cases (28.3%) were improved—i.e., able to sleep five to six hours; and only one case (2.2%) failed—i.e., able to sleep less than three hours. The **success rate was 97.8%**.

- **Immune response** against infection

- **Depression**, anxiety and other mental disorders

- **Recovery from paralysis**

- **Alcoholism:** A study of chronic alcoholics found that subjects who participated in a trial of auriculotherapy had **50% less drinking episodes**, and 50% less return visits to detoxification facilities, compared with a control group.

- **Diabetes mellitus**

- **Sinusitis**

- **Bronchitis**

- **Cold and flu symptoms**
- **Gastrointestinal disorders** such as Crohn's Disease
- **The correction of imbalances** in the body and a wide variety of health conditions originating from every bodily system.

For many people, auriculotherapy is also the treatment of choice for **eliminating addictive behaviors** including *alcohol and drug abuse* (street and recreational drugs), attention deficit disorder, obsessive-compulsive disorder, and even gambling.

Auriculotherapy is similar to ear acupuncture but instead of using needles, a microcurrent stimulator is placed on reflex points on the outer ear. These points then send a message to the brain based on the location of the reflex point being treated.

There are various modes of auriculotherapy administration, including sonopuncture (ultrasound), laser therapy, electro-acupuncture and piezo electric acupuncture stimulator. But by far, the simplest mode of auriculotherapy administration is through **ear acupressure** (also called ear reflexology), which utilizes finger pressure, or a narrow, blunt-tipped wand, such as the end of a match stick.

Once you learn how to *identify the reflex points on the outer ear that have a therapeutic effect on the body* (such as the point for **Appetite Control**, the **Anti-Depressant** point, the **Insomnia point**, the **Smoking Cessation** point), and discover the simple technique for stimulating those points, you'll be able to employ the *do-it-yourself approach* at home.

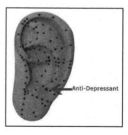

Ear acupressure is a method that requires the use of your fingers (or simple paraphernalia, such as herbal beads, pellets or a blunt wand) to apply pressure on the reflex points (also referred to as auricular points). Although this method is very simple, it can nonetheless, help you experience the therapeutic benefits mentioned above—without needles, micro-current, special equipment, or a visit to a health practitioner who specializes in auriculotherapy.

Health Benefits (and Other Little-Known Amazing Effects) of Auriculotherapy

Since the outer ear is a *microsystem* that connects to every part of the human body, auriculotherapy relieves a wide variety of health problems. Virtually all health conditions can be improved to some degree by stimulating the ear points.

Many practitioners of *Qi Gong*, an internal Chinese healing art that promotes the circulation of *qi* (pronounced *chee*), or vital energy, within the human body, make it a daily practice to massage their ears as a way of *enhancing overall health*. Traditional Chinese medicine believes that pain, disease, or dysfunction is due to a blockage of qi within the body. The stimulation of ear acupuncture points is believed to help restore the normal flow of qi, thereby relieving symptoms that resulted from its stagnation or blockage.

To learn more about *The Amazing Science of Auriculotherapy*, go to: http://undergroundhealthreporter.com/the-amazing-science-of-auriculotherapy

Chapter 15 - You Can Win the "Battle of the Bulge"

The Top Three Myths Propagated by Weight Management "Experts" that Could Make You Obese and Unhealthy

Obesity rates are rising at an alarming rate. Americans are getting fatter and fatter, with obesity rates reaching 30 percent or more in nine states last year, as opposed to only three states in 2007.[12]

According to Dr. Thomas Frieden, Director of the Centers for Disease Control and Prevention, obesity rates have **doubled in adults** and **tripled in children** in recent decades. This makes obesity one of America's most pressing health problems.

At the time of this writing, 72.5 million people—that is, **26.7% of Americans** are obese! An additional 34% are overweight. Global statistics show that over 300 million people in the world are diagnosed as clinically obese.

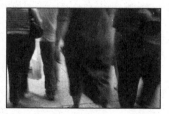

People over the age of 50 have higher rates of obesity than those who are younger, according to Dr. Heidi Blanck, Chief of the CDC's obesity branch.

If you (or your children) are obese or just weigh too much, the lack of physical activity is only part of the problem. The food industry is bent on encouraging the consumption of supersized portions of high-fat, high-sugar foods.

Furthermore, even so-called fitness experts unknowingly disseminate health advice that not only makes you *unhealthy*, but actually makes you

---

[12] Managing Editor, *The Underground Health Reporter*

fatter. Here are the Top Three Myths propagated by weight management experts:

Myth No. 1: Eat proteins and carbohydrates at every meal.

"Experts" would have you believe that you must consume glucose, glycogen or carbohydrates in order to transport and digest proteins properly. That's why most suggested menus featured in practically all weight management programs (except low-carb and no-carb programs) recommend a serving of protein and a serving of carbohydrate in the same meal. For example, meat and potatoes, fish and rice, etc.

This is totally untrue. The basic concept is correct—i.e., the only way protein can build muscle is when it is consumed with adequate amounts of carbohydrates. The *mistake* is that they advise people to consume proteins and carbohydrates in the same meal.

Eating proteins together with carbohydrates is actually **counterproductive to weight loss** because it takes different amounts of time to digest proteins and carbs. For example, it takes longer to digest meat than fruit. Therefore, it is unwise to eat them together because:

> The fruit only takes about 20 to 30 minutes to digest, and then moves on to the small intestines. It remains there with the meat, which takes three or more hours to digest, causing the food to ferment. The fermented food then travels to the colon, where it sits even longer and begins to *putrefy*. According to a recent U.S. survey, an average American male has about **5 pounds of undigested, putrefied red meat** in his stomach at any given time, and incomplete digestion is one of the prime causes of fat accumulation in the body.

Even common sense will tell you that no matter what kind of diet plan you follow, carrying around that extra weight won't be beneficial to your weight management goals (not to mention your health) if your food is undigested, or poorly digested at best.

Over time, this inferior mode of eating also causes the colon to become overly toxic, and, because it overburdens the digestive glands, it produces health problems including digestive stress, gas, heartburn, cramps, bloating, constipation, foul stool, bleeding piles, colitis—and even **colon cancer**.

According to Dr. Suzanne Gudakunst, **the only doctor who has found a cure for obesity**, proper food combining involves *eating foods that have the same digestion times* in the same meal. For optimum digestion and assimilation, she advises, **"Eat protein and starch/carbohydrates SEPARATELY."**

Myth No. 2: Eat a high-protein diet

Ask any Hollywood star who has lost a lot of pounds, what they did to shed so much weight and one of the things they're likely to tell you is that their fitness trainer told them to eat huge amounts of protein—usually in the form of **egg whites**, chicken, turkey, lean steaks and burgers, fish, etc.

When it comes to building muscle, it's true that nothing is more important than getting the right amount of protein. That's because a diet rich in protein has been shown to raise one's Resting Metabolic Rate by as much as 68%. So just by eating protein, you immediately speed up your metabolism, thereby enabling your body to increase lean muscle mass and decrease body fat faster.

However, regular over-consumption of protein leads to excessive **dehydration**, as well as **toxicity** of the liver, kidneys and brain. Many fitness "gurus," personal trainers and protein supplement marketers would have you believe that you need at least one gram of protein per pound of body weight. That's ill-conceived advice—often, just pure marketing.

The recommended protein intake that is *scientifically* proven to increase muscle mass is 0.8 grams of protein per kilogram (or 2.2 pounds) of body weight. That's **0.36 grams of protein per pound of body weight per day**. This also happens to be the U.S. government's recommended dietary allowance (RDA).

The **quality of protein** you consume is also paramount. Most protein sources, such as meat and dairy, are acid-forming. One of the best ways to maintain weight loss is to **minimize the consumption of acid-forming foods**.

"When you change your food choices to alkaline, your body becomes a fat-burning machine and prevents many diseases," says Dr. Gudakunst. She recommends an eating plan that consists of **80% alkaline-forming foods and 20% acid-forming foods**.

Also, to counteract the dehydration that high protein consumption produces, you should consume more water. To figure out how much water to drink, Dr. Gudakunst says, "Take your body weight and divide it by two —and that is the amount of water in ounces that you should be drinking each day."

If you do nothing else but drink your recommended amount of water, you will accelerate your results—sometimes by **two to four additional pounds**—or more—**lost** per month. The only downside to drinking the recommended amount of water is frequent urination. But remember that every single time you urinate, you're getting rid of ugly fat, as well as unwanted waste and toxins.

Myth No. 3: Exercise for at least 30 minutes in order to burn body fat

Fitness enthusiasts always insist that for any exercise to burn fat, it must be done for at least 30 minutes. They point to research that shows that only after 30 minutes of exercise does the body begin to use its stored glycogen. And only after the body burns the stored glycogen does it start burning fat.

This time-consuming way of exercising is not only antiquated, it also rarely produces rapid results. This news may come as a shock to people who religiously spend 30 to 60 minutes doing aerobics or using treadmills, rowing machines, ellipticals and other exercise equipment several times a week in an effort to lose body fat. These types of time-intensive workouts usually result in only 0.2 pound of fat lost per week. That's only *one-fifth of one pound of fat lost* after all that time and effort.

Instead of the old-fashioned way of working out, Dr. Gudakunst recommends **brief bursts of anaerobic exercise**. She says, "Intense anaerobic exercise stimulates the production of growth hormone, which is **a strong stimulator of fat burning**."

Furthermore, when you exercise at high-intensity levels, your body burns fat through a process known as the Krebs cycle. The Krebs cycle is what metabolizes fat into energy. The duration of the high-intensity exercise must necessarily be brief because that's when the body calls on its stored fat, and turns that fat into fuel for energy. If you do the exercise for much longer periods, your body will start to burn glucose. Glucose then becomes the fuel of choice, and your body will begin to **devour muscle tissue** and convert it to glucose for energy.

A short-duration, high-intensity anaerobic exercise **turns your body into a mega fat-burning furnace** that will burn fat not only during, but well after you perform the exercise. It achieves better results than 45 to 60 minutes of aerobic or cardiovascular workouts like walking or jogging.

In her book, *Top Secret Fat Loss Secret*, Dr. Suzanne Gudakunst reveals the No. 1 reason why most people can't lose weight permanently—it has nothing to do with will power, over-eating or the right diet. It has to do with the plaque and harmful parasites that exist in your colon. Once you get rid of them, you can easily shed 10, 25, 50 pounds—even 100 pounds or more.

To read our article on the top 3 weight loss myths and discover the scientifically proven way to shed weight and keep it off for good go to http://undergroundhealthreporter.com/shed-weight-for-good

Georgetown Study: A Compound that Blocks Carbs Also Burns Fat

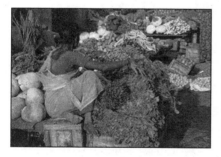

Georgetown University in Washington, DC conducted an eight-week study focused on a *curious Asian fruit* that grows in India and Indonesia. There's a unique compound in the rind of this fruit, which has the remarkable ability to block the enzyme in your body that turns carbs into fat.

By blocking this enzyme, the compound helps your body use carbs more efficiently—and makes your appetite disappear.

Here are the results of the Georgetown Universit study in which 60 people participated:

➢ Significant *decrease* in:

  • Total body weight

  • Total food intake

> Significant *increase* in:

- Serotonin (the "feel good" brain chemical)

- Fat oxidation (fat burning)

- Cardiovascular benefits

A Mineral that Burns Fat

As if the compound used in the Georgetown study weren't enough, the researchers took another **extraordinary** mineral and combined it with the compound from the Asian fruit. Here are the details of just one study involving this mineral.

Dr. Gil Kaats and a team of researchers from the Health and Medical Research Foundation and the University of Texas Health Science Center studied over 150 people to see if they would lose fat just from taking this mineral alone.

They split the 150 participants into 3 groups: one group received a placebo (an inert sugar pill); the other two groups received the mineral. The participants were told not to change anything else in their diet, or their exercise habits or in how much they ate. In essence, they were allowed to do whatever they wanted.

After three months, the group taking the placebo showed no changes. The participants in the groups that received the mineral **lost between 3.4 and 4.6 pounds of body fat**—and they also **gained an average of 1.4 pounds of pure muscle**. That's from making absolutely no changes—except taking the mineral daily.

Dr. Al Sears has perfected a formula that combines these two nutrients with yet another exotic, all-natural fat-burning herb (also an excellent appetite suppressant) from the Kalahari Desert. In so doing, he's developed a **revolutionary recipe for weight loss** and the prevention and reduction of obesity.

The formula is administered via a unique delivery system—you simply spray it into your mouth. Just two sprays are sufficient, and the fat burning, appetite suppressing effect lasts for hours.

Shed Pounds and Lower Cholesterol with this Exotic Fruit Extract

The Wellness Research Foundation in Royal Palm Beach has recently discovered a formula that may well become known as the pivotal discovery in man's never-ending battle of the "bulge." The formula consists of a fruit extract from the jungles of West Africa and a seaweed from Japan.

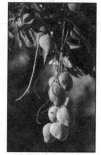

The first part of the proprietary formula is a fruit extract obtained from the African mango (*Irvingia gabonensis*). Fox News reports: "Lab research has shown that extracts from the plant's seed may **inhibit body fat production**, through effects on certain genes and enzymes that **regulate metabolism**."

Researchers at the University of Yaounde in Cameroon conducted a randomized, placebo-controlled study of 102 overweight adults and placed them in two groups—one group taking the fruit extract, and the other group taking a placebo—twice a day for ten weeks. The study participants were not required to follow any special diet and were instructed to maintain their normal exercise levels.

By the end of the study, the group that received the fruit extract had **lost an average of 28 pounds** while the placebo group showed almost no change. It was also found that the "bad" LDL cholesterol and blood sugar levels of those in the control group declined significantly. These findings were published in the online journal *Lipids in Health and Disease*.

However, it wasn't until the Wellness Research Foundation combined the fruit extract with an extract from the Japanese seaweed (Undaria pinnatifida) that truly remarkable results were seen.

A Microscopic Protein that Burns Fat While You're Resting!

The seaweed extract contains an ingredient called *fucoxanthin*. When a group of Japanese marine biologists fed their study animals with fucoxanthin, *something remarkable happened*: A microscopic protein—called UCP1—suddenly became active.

189

This protein turns up your metabolic furnace and lets your cells burn fat for energy—not during exercise, but **while you're resting**. This safe and nutritious seaweed extract actually flips your metabolic switch and "turns on" your body's fat-burning machinery.

WRF's formula consisting of both the fruit extract from the African mango and the extract from the Japanese seaweed appears to have a synergistic effect that may quite possibly be the **easiest and most potent way to drop pounds and fat**. Some of the extraordinary results seen by users of the formula are the effortless shedding of fat (especially **belly fat**), a leaner and tighter stomach, suppression of hunger and appetite, diminished food cravings, increased energy levels, fast loss of two or more women's dress sizes and up to **75 pounds of unwanted weight lost within six months**.

A Mushroom that Makes You Skinny

Many health-conscious people have already discovered that the medicinal reishi mushroom has **extraordinary health- and longevity enhancing properties,** is a *super immune booster*—and is one of the most powerful herbs known to man. What most people don't know is that **Reishi mushrooms can also make you skinny**, or help eliminate unwanted weight.

Dr. Suzanne Gudakunst, the doctor who recently **discovered the cure for obesity**—much to the consternation of the medical and food industries that make billions of dollars by keeping people fat—developed a proprietary method of dehydrating Reishi mushrooms down to a tiny fraction of their size, and encase them in a small capsule. When you take the capsule (called Skinny Shrooms) as directed, the reishi mushroom expands in your stomach. This not only makes you feel full, it goes further than that.

The feeling of *satiety* (which tells your body, "I am full" and to stop eating) does not come from your stomach. It comes from your brain. Some experts say it takes an average of twenty minutes for the body's signal to reach the brain. This is what usually causes weight gain. If you eat an entire meal in less than twenty minutes, you would have consumed hundreds of calories more than your body really wants before the satiety signal makes it to the brain.

With the reishi mushroom capsule, you don't have to rely on the feeling of fullness produced in your stomach to reach your brain, it actually **activates the satiety response** (which originates in the hypothalamus) that tells you to stop eating.

In addition, because reishi mushrooms are a nutrient-dense "super food"—and not just a dietary supplement—they actually provide super nutrition that most diets never provide.

What Fitness and Nutrition "Gurus" Won't Tell You

All major diets—whether it is the South Beach Diet, the Atkins, Zone or Master Cleanse diet—DO work. But only for a *little while*.

It doesn't take a genius to know that if you cut down your carbohydrate intake (as recommended by the Atkins Diet) or you go on a lemonade diet for ten days—or replace two meals a day with Slimfast, Special K or a protein drink and have just one sensible dinner thereafter—you WILL lose weight.

But a weight loss program is only truly effective if it works with—and not against—the natural biochemistry of the human body and if it promotes good health.

What good is a high-protein diet that makes you gain muscle and lose fat if it causes toxicity of the liver, kidneys and brain? Yes, that's what a high-protein diet does to you in the long run.

What good is it if you got really skinny on a low-fat diet, but the diet causes your skin to sag and hang loosely, or ovarian cysts (in women) and low sperm or testosterone counts (in men)? Yes, that's what a low-fat diet does. Have you ever noticed that most weight management "experts" look haggard and old for their age?

What good is a diet that has the 40-30-30 balance of macronutrients if it causes constant digestive distress? And what good is having a lean, great-looking body if the process of acquiring it causes you to be in poor health?

Dr. Gudakunst's *Skinny Shrooms* can, once and for all, enable you to lose unwanted pounds while honoring your body's nutritional needs so that you can keep the weight off forever—and you won't jeopardize your health in the process of shedding pounds. This is what most so-called fitness and nutrition gurus won't tell you.

No More Food Cravings

Another **secret mechanism** at work in Skinny Shrooms is that reishi mushrooms "mineralize" your body, causing **food cravings to virtually disappear**. It is a well-known scientific fact that mineral deficiencies (such as a deficiency in chromium and vanadium) cause sugar cravings and other fattening predispositions.

In addition to effective weight management, Dr. Gudakunst's Skinny Shrooms comes with all the health benefits of reishi mushrooms, which have been used in Traditional Chinese Medicine for more than 4,000 years.

Among the most common health issues treated with this herbal relief are:

- Inflammatory Disease like Arthritis, Colitis, etc.
- Asthma
- Nervous Disorders
- High Blood Pressure
- Cancer Tumors
- High Cholesterol
- Allergies
- Mononucleosis
- Chronic Infections
- Hepatitis

A high quality reishi mushroom supplement in tablet or capsule form costs upwards of $50.00 a bottle. And although that reishi supplement might provide excellent nutritional support, it won't be in Dr. Gudakunst's proprietary dehydrated form that expands in your stomach, activates the satiety response in the brain and makes you skinny. Skinny Shrooms cost only a fraction of what reishi supplements normally cost. Dr. Gudakunst is letting readers of this book **get a ten-day supply completely free of charge**. All you have to pay is a small shipping charge. Simply go to the following webpage, scroll down the page and click on the "Order Now" button: http://undergroundhealthreporter.com/skinnyshrooms01

Don't Fall for the *Acai* Berry "Tiny Belly" Trick — Here's What Really Works

They seem to be everywhere—those banner advertisements on the Internet that have headlines like: "#1 Trick of a Tiny Belly" or "The #1 Best Tip for Getting a Flat Belly," which always seem to be accompanied by the animated graphic of a woman's body shrinking from fat to thin.

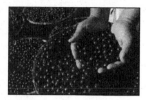

If you've ever tried clicking on those banner ads, you probably discovered that the advertisers are promoting their respective brands of acai berry juice or supplements. *Acai* berries are apparently the key that's *supposed* to create a flat belly.

Acai berries (pronounced ah-SAH'-ee) definitely have numerous health properties, and are considered a "super fruit" with remarkable antioxidant content. However, their ability to trim belly fat is **dubious**. In addition, Internet marketers selling acai berries often are illegally claiming that Oprah Winfrey endorsed acai berries. They are willfully using the names of celebrities and well-known figures to deceive the public. Oprah vehemently denies these marketers' claims.

Oprah Files a Trademark Infringement Complaint Against 40 Internet Marketers

Oprah Winfrey's website, Oprah.com, states that:

On August 19, 2009, Harpo, Inc., producers of The Oprah Winfrey Show and The Dr. Oz Show, along with Dr. Mehmet Oz, filed a trademark infringement complaint against 40 Internet marketers of dietary supplements, including acai berry products among others. Neither Ms. Winfrey nor Dr. Oz has ever sponsored or endorsed any acai berry ... dietary supplement product.

Drinking acai berry juice (or any other fruit juice, for that matter) adds sugar to your diet. And sugar from any source—be it from sugar cane or beet, corn syrup, and, yes, even fruit **causes fat to accumulate in your belly**.

193

Consuming more than fifteen grams of sugar on any given day affects the amount of insulin in your body. Insulin is a hormone produced by your pancreas to manage your blood sugar and control the accumulation of fat, especially belly fat. Insulin is referred to as "the primary regulator of fat tissue."

Therefore, even if you think you're doing yourself a favor by drinking acai berry juice, the increased level of insulin that the sugar in the juice produces will make you fat and make sure you stay fat.

The same is true of any juice diet, such as the Celebrity Juice Diet—and even the Master Cleanse diet, which consists of lemon juice, cayenne pepper and Grade B maple syrup (sugar!). It's easy to see why such diets would make you drop pounds because they obviously lack of calories and flush your system. However, the weight you'll lose is primarily water weight, and once you revert to your old eating habits, the pounds will return.

So many diet myths like these abound, and it's often difficult to know which fat loss diets actually work—and which ones are actually counter-productive to your fat loss goals.

Discover the REAL trick for getting a tiny belly from a man who actually **lost 42 pounds of fat and ten inches off his belly in just a few weeks**—and whose wife **lost nearly 60 pounds and eight dress sizes** at the same time. There is an informative video that shows you how easily they did it. It is definitely eye-opening, whether you're someone who wants to lose only your belly fat—or someone who wants to rid your entire body of fat.

The video can be found at:
http://undergroundhealthreporter.com/tinybellytrick

Epilogue

1-½ Cent Healthcare for Recessionary Times

If you're worried about the **alarming** impact that the new healthcare Law will have on your life, you have every reason to be concerned.

We're living in uncertain economic times, and the new healthcare law has brought forth even more questions than answers.

> ➤ How much higher will healthcare costs rise as a result of the new law?
>
> ➤ Will you be able to afford your health insurance premiums if they go up by 30% to 45%?
>
> ➤ What will you do if there comes a time when you can no longer rely on Medicare or Social Security—because they are broke?
>
> ➤ Where can you turn if doctors and hospitals turn you away because they have no assurance they'll get paid for the services they provide to you?

If you're an American over the age of 40—or if you have parents or family members who are retirees or are close to retirement age, you MUST take the necessary steps right now to protect yourself from the coming healthcare crisis.

The repercussions of the new healthcare law may not be evident now, but they will become the sobering reality in the next few years.

The *good news* is that there is a 1½ cent solution to your healthcare worries. You can get the details in a free 5-minute video titled *"1½ Cent Healthcare for Recessionary Times."*

Don't wait until the year 2014 (when the full effect of the healthcare Law is unleashed) before taking action. If you wait till then, you will never be sure if your healthcare needs will be met. Nor will you have any control over whether or not you will receive healthcare benefits from the government—or how much your insurance will cost you.

Read *"1½ Cent Healthcare for Recessionary Times"* now by going to: http://www.1minutecure.com/index-OneAndAHalfCentHealthcare.htm, and don't forget to send this link to everyone you know. Every family must read this article.

Index

Anderson, Craig 139
Anderson, Mike 23
anthocyanins 13
Anthrax 45
anti-amyloid 37
antibiotics 9, 25, 34, 43-44, 59, 63-64,
    after-effects of 43
    resistance to 43, 64
    types of 43
antibodies 24, 62, 80
Anticancer Research (journal) 165
anti-carcinogenics 38
anticoagulants 13
anti-inflammatory 9, 25, 37, 73-74, 98-99,
114, 117, 167
anti-malignin antibodies (AMAs) 23-24
    detecting and measuring 23
Anti Malignan Antibody in Serum
(AMAS) test 23
    accuracy of 24
    clinical support for 24
    Oncolab home test kit for 24
antioxidatives/antioxidants 9, 11-13, 16,
25, 33, 37-39, 49, 60-62, 72-73, 97-98,
117-118, 123,
    health risks; high doses of 97-98
    false hypothesis about 97-98
antipyretics (fever reducing) 98
aphrodisiac (see sexual attraction)
Aspirin 69, 80, 94, 98-99, 167
anxiety 6, 16, 31, 72-73, 79, 145, 150,
173, 176, 180
apoptosis/apoptosis mechanism; cancer
cell self-destruction 27
argyria 44-45
arteries; thickening of 49, 60, 88, 137
    preventing 90, 139
arthritis 14, 18, 31-34, 40, 72-74, 92-94,
98-99, 112, 114, 127-130, 145, 150, 192
    causes of joint pain in 127, 130
    halting cartilage breakdown 130-131
    non-surgical joint replacement 127-
131
    risks of prescription medications for
(see also NSAIDs) 98-100

arthritis (continued)
    traditional treatments for 127-128
        effectiveness of 127-128, 130
ascorbic acid (see vitamin C)
Asmanex 87
Asthma 9, 16, 31, 87-88, 192
    prescription medicine 87
        side effects; localized 87
        side effects; systemic 87
    vitamin D insufficiency and 87-88
atoms 95
athlete's foot 34, 64
Atkins Diet 191
ATP (adenosine triphosphate) 6
auriculotherapy (see alternative medicine)
autism 40, 155
auxin/ auxinon 15
    foods rich in 15
Avian Influenza (H5N1)
avobenzone (parsol 1789) 164
avocado (persea gratissima; p. americana;
alligator pear) 57-59
    nutritional benefits of 57-58
    servings suggestions for 58-59
Awakening Prologue CD (Bill Harris)
175-178
Ayurvedic medicine 25, 37-39, 162
AZT (azidothymidine) 36

B

bacillus subtilis 88
bacteria 23, 34, 42-44, 59-61, 63-64, 73,
88-89, 92-93, 95-96
    "good" forms of 19, 44, 89
    pathogenic/ anaerobic 44
    staphylococcus 64
    "zapping" away (see Zapper)
Bannister, Roger 151
Barron, Jon 166-167
Beals, Dr. Paul 112-113
bee pollen 8-11
    cautions in use of 11
    clinical support for 9-11
    dosage recommendations for 10-11
    forms of 10

juice 10, 12-13, 20-21, 30, 40, 65-66, 193
juicing; versus blending 65-66

K

Kaats, Dr. Gil 188
kalpa vriksha (see coconut)
Karason, Paul 44
Kay, Dr. Neil 146
Khalsa, Karta Purkh Singh 37, 39
Khan, Chaka 179-180
Ketoprofen (orudis KT) 99, 167
Kennedy, Dr. Ron 92, 94
kidneys 7, 11, 20, 28-29, 41, 107, 167,
185, 191
    damage 191
Kleiser, Grenville 141
Kodama, Dr. Noriko 47
kombu (laminaria japonica/brown
seaweed), see brown seaweed
Komuta, Dr. Kiyoshi 47
konnyaku (konjac) potato
(Amorphophallus konjac/devil's tongue)
104-105
    cautions in use of
    dosage recommendations for 105
    forms of 105
    health benefits of 104-105
    historical medicinal use of 104
    sources for purchasing 105
kola nut 7
Kupfer, Dr. Carl 122

L

La Chi; Qigong exercise 31-32
Lam, Dr. Michael 74
laminaria japonica (see brown seaweed)
laminarin 27, 29
Lananki, Antti 10
Lancet, The 99
Landone, Dr. Brown 15
Landy, John 153
Langager, Stacy 146
Learning Strategies 155, 173
Leavitt, Dr. Ron 43

lecithin (also see soy lecithin) 139
    importance of 139
lentinan 35-36
lepidium meyenii (see maca)
leukotriene modifiers 87
Li, Ching-Yun 5, 12
Li, Shizhen 7
Libido 9, 11, 71, 180
lipiodol (iodized poppy seed oil) 47
Lipitor 90
Lipton, Dr. Bruce 54-55, 152
liver 7, 11, 16, 19, 21, 28-29, 35, 38, 41,
48, 63, 69, 112, 139, 147, 167, 185, 191
    detoxification of 19, 21, 28, 63
    liver failure, acute (see
    acetaminophen)
Los Angeles Times, The 159, 169
Lou Gehrig's Disease 150
love, healing effects of 51-53
Loyd, Dr. Alex 149-150
Lu, Dr. Yan Fang 31
Luks, Allan 79
lutein 58
LuvEssentials 172
lycium barbarum (see goji berry)
lymphatic system 78

M

maca (lepidium meyenii) 71-72
    nutritional benefits of 71-72
    therapeutic uses of 71-72
macular degeneration 11, 58, 122-123
    age-related (AMD) 122
    blindness resulting from 122
Mae, Dr. Tatsumasa 124
magnesium (see minerals)
Main, Dr. Bart 148
mainstream medicine 96, 132, 135, 140,
151
maitake mushroom (grifola frondosa)
46-48
    cancer fighting properties of 46-48
    case studies using 7-48
    clinical support for 46
    forms of 48

If you enjoyed this book
and wish to learn more health secrets
and little-known health discoveries,
subscribe to the Underground Health Reporter™
e-newsletter for FREE at
www.UndergroundHealthReporter.com

√ Order copies to give away
to friends and family members by going to
http://www.UndergroundHealthReporter.com/order.htm

√ To order our other book titles, go to
http://www.ThinkOutsideTheBook.com

or contact
Think-Outside-the-Book Publishing, LLC
8484 Wilshire Boulevard, Suite 760
Beverly Hills, CA 90211

(800) 665-4732